The Complete
Zero Point Weight Loss
Cookbook

1200 days of quick weight loss and long-term health include tasty, easy-to-make recipes.

Justin Rock

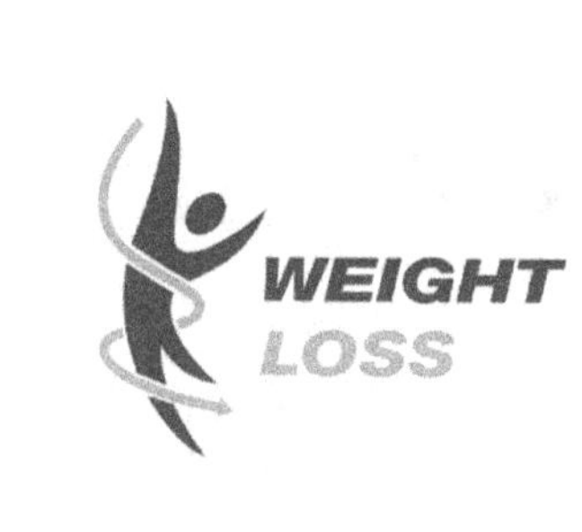

Copyright © 2024 by Justin Rock

All rights reserved. No portion of this book may be reproduced in any form without permission from the publisher, except as permitted by U.S. copyright law. For permissions contact with author.

<u>LEGAL NOTICE</u>

The copyright for this work has been secured. This book is intended for individual study alone. Without the express written permission of the author-publisher, you may not alter, copy, sell, use, quote, or paraphrase any of the material included herein in any form.

<u>DISCLAIMER NOTICE</u>

This document is intended solely for your use, education, and enjoyment. We have ensured that the data presented here is correct. No express or implied guarantees are made. The reader understands that the author does not render professional, medical, legal, or financial advice. This book's contents were compiled from a wide range of resources. Before attempting any of the methods discussed here, you should get the advice of a qualified expert.

Table of Contents:

INTRODUCTION_

Welcome to "The Complete Zero Point Weight Loss Cookbook," a complete guide that will help you lose weight while still eating tasty, filling meals. The ideas in this cookbook come from the idea of "zero point foods," which were made popular by weight loss programs like Weight Watchers. These foods are given zero points because they are low in calories and high in nutrients. These foods are the building blocks of a healthy, well-balanced diet, and you don't have to carefully track every calorie when you eat them.

There are recipes for breakfast, lunch, dinner, snacks, and even sweets in this cookbook. There is something for everyone to enjoy, from rich desserts and tasty main dishes to colorful salads and hearty soups.

This cookbook has tasty recipes that are also very simple to make because they use common ingredients and give clear instructions. You'll find a lot of ideas for satisfying meals that will help you reach your weight loss goals, no matter how much or how little cooking experience you have.

Along with tasty recipes, this cookbook gives you good advice on how to include "zero-point" foods in your daily meals. You'll learn how to make well-balanced meals, pick healthy foods, and stay on track when you're with other people or eating out.

The Complete Zero Point Weight Loss Cookbook will take you on a tasty and healthy food adventure. This cookbook will help you make healthier choices, lose weight, and live your best life by giving you a lot of tasty recipes and useful tips. Let's start cooking!

THE CONCEPT OF ZERO POINT FOODS

Most zero-point foods are high in nutrients and low in calories, which makes them an important part of a healthy diet. Some low-fat dairy products, fruits, and vegetables are among them. These foods were chosen because they make you feel full, are good for you, and are less likely to make you eat too much. Focusing on foods with no points lets you eat more without hurting your weight loss efforts.

WHY ZERO POINT FOODS WORK

Zero-point foods are meant to help people eat healthier by focusing on foods that are naturally lower in calories but higher in fiber, vitamins, and minerals. These foods keep you full longer, which makes you less likely to snack on unhealthy foods. You can also focus on the quality of your food instead of the quantity since you won't have to count points for these foods.

BENEFITS OF THE ZERO POINT APPROACH

1. *Simplifies Meal Planning:* When you have zero-point foods, it's easier to plan your meals. You don't have to keep track of every bite because you can mix and match these foods to make a wide range of satisfying meals.

2. *Promotes Nutrient-Dense Eating:* Zero-point foods are full of important nutrients that help you eat in a way that is good for your health as a whole.

3. *Encourages Healthy Habits:* By focusing on fruits, vegetables, lean proteins, and other healthy foods, you'll naturally start eating better, which can help you lose weight and keep it off.

4. *Reduces Food Anxiety:* Having a list of foods that you can eat whenever you want without going against your progress can help you feel less stressed about dieting and food choices.

WHAT TO EXPECT FROM THIS COOKBOOK

"The Complete Zero Point Weight Loss Cookbook" is the best way to find healthy, tasty meals that will help you lose weight. You'll find the following inside:

- **A Variety of Recipes:** This cookbook has a lot of different recipes for breakfast, lunch, dinner, and snacks that all use zero-point foods as their main ingredients.
- **Easy-to-Follow Instructions:** It's easy for cooks of all levels to make healthy meals because each recipe is meant to be clear and simple.
- **Nutritional Information:** The focus is on foods with no points, and each recipe has nutrition facts to help you keep track of what you're eating.
- **Meal Planning Tips:** To make a healthy, enjoyable eating plan, learn how to plan your meals around foods that count as zero points.
- **Weight Loss Support:** This cookbook has recipes as well as advice on how to stay motivated and on track with your weight loss plans.

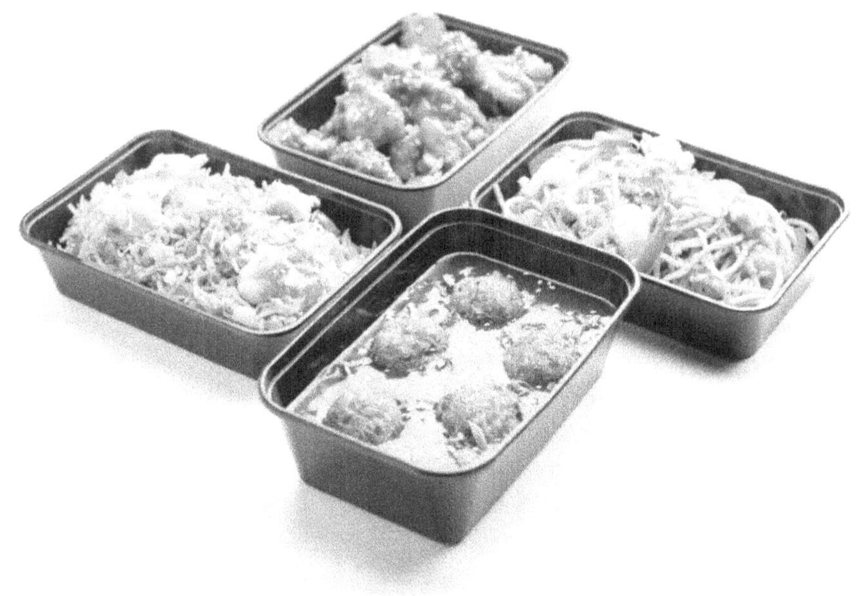

EMBRACING A ZERO POINT LIFESTYLE

A zero-point approach to eating isn't just a way to lose weight; it's also a way to make long-term changes that will help you live a healthier life. The goal of this cookbook is to help you discover the joy of cooking and eating tasty, healthy meals that make you feel full and energized. You can make progress toward your weight loss goals and keep a healthy relationship with food by eating foods that don't count against you.

"The Complete Zero Point Weight Loss Cookbook" is here to help you on your way, whether you're new to the idea of zero-point foods or just want some new ideas. As you change the way you eat and your life, enjoy the process, enjoy the tastes, and be proud of your progress.

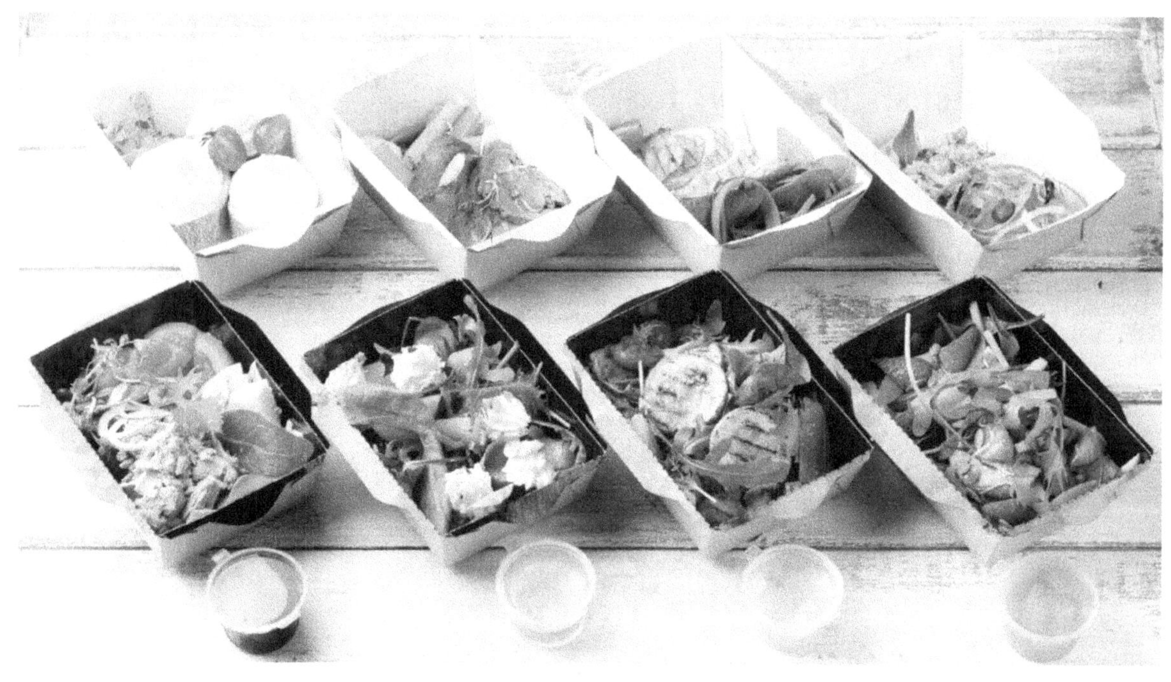

BREAKFAST RECIPES

Avocado Toast

Prep Time: 5 minutes

Cook Time: 5 minutes

Servings: 2

Ingredients:

- 2 ripe avocados
- 4 slices of whole grain bread
- 1 lemon
- Salt and pepper to taste
- Optional toppings: cherry tomatoes, red pepper flakes, feta cheese, poached egg

Instructions:

1. Brown the pieces of whole grain bread in the oven until they're browned.
2. In the meanwhile, cut the avocados in half and scoop out the pits. Place the avocado flesh in a bowl using a spoon.
3. Use a fork to mash the avocado until it becomes smooth.
4. Add half a lemon's juice to the mashed avocado and stir to combine. Taste and add salt and pepper as needed.
5. Evenly distribute the mashed avocado over the toasted bread.
6. Add whatever toppings you want on top.
7. Quickly prepare and enjoy!

Nutrition Information (per serving): Calories: ~250, Fat: ~15g, Carbohydrates: ~25g, Protein: ~5g

Smoked Salmon Bagel

Prep Time: 10 minutes

Cook Time: N/A (No cooking required)

Servings: 2

Ingredients:

- 2 bagels, sliced and toasted
- 4 oz. smoked salmon
- 4 oz. cream cheese
- 1 small red onion, thinly sliced
- Capers (optional)
- Fresh dill (optional)
- Lemon wedges (optional)

Instructions:

1. On top of the toasted bagel

slices, spread the cream cheese equally.
2. On top of the cream cheese, arrange slices of smoked salmon.
3. Arrange some red onion slices on the smoked salmon.
4. If preferred, garnish with capers and fresh dill.
5. Accompany the dish with slices of lemon.
6. Those smoked salmon bagels are very mouthwatering.

Nutrition Information (per serving): Calories: ~400, Fat: ~15g, Carbohydrates: ~45g, Protein: ~20g

Berry Smoothie Bowl

Prep Time: 5 minutes

Cook Time: 0 minutes

Servings: 1

Ingredients:

- 1 frozen banana
- 1 cup of mixed berries (such as strawberries, blueberries, raspberries)
- ½ cup of plain Greek yogurt
- ¼ cup of almond milk
- Toppings: granola, sliced fruits, shredded coconut, chia seeds, honey

Instructions:

1. Frozen banana, mixed berries, Greek yogurt, and almond milk should all be blended together.
2. Add more almond milk as required to get the desired consistency, and blend until the mixture is smooth and creamy.
3. Fill a bowl with the smoothie.
4. Add granola, fruit slices, coconut flakes, chia seeds, and honey, or anything you choose.
5. Indulge in your luscious berry smoothie bowl right now!

Nutrition Information (per serving): Calories: ~300, Fat: ~5g, Carbohydrates: ~55g, Protein: ~15g

Banana Pancakes

Prep Time: 10 minutes

Cook Time: 10 minutes

Servings: 2-3

Ingredients:

- 2 ripe bananas, mashed
- 2 eggs
- ½ cup of oat flour (you can make your own by blending oats)
- 1 **tsp** baking powder
- ½ **tsp** vanilla extract
- Pinch of salt
- Butter or oil for cooking
- Optional toppings: sliced bananas, berries, maple syrup, nut butter

Instructions:

1. Mash the ripe bananas until they are completely smooth in a mixing basin with a fork.
2. Incorporate the mashed bananas with the eggs, oat flour, baking powder, vanilla essence, and a dash of salt. Whisk until well blended.
3. Sauté some butter or oil in a nonstick pan or griddle set over medium heat.
4. For every pancake, add a quarter cup of batter to the pan.
5. Turnover and cook for another two to three minutes, or until golden brown.
6. If the pan needs extra oil or butter, add more. Repeat with the rest of the batter.
7. Toppings like sliced bananas, berries, maple syrup, and nut butter are perfect for these warm pancakes.
8. Slurp up those delicious banana pancakes!

Nutrition Information (per serving, based on 2 servings):

Calories: ~250, Fat: ~8g, Carbohydrates: ~35g, Protein: ~9g

Veggie Frittata

Prep Time: 15 minutes

Cook Time: 25 minutes

Servings: 4

Ingredients:

- 8 eggs
- ¼ cup of milk (dairy or plant-based)
- 1 cup of chopped vegetables (such as bell peppers, onions, spinach, mushrooms)
- ½ cup of grated cheese (such as cheddar, mozzarella, or feta)
- Salt and pepper to taste
- 1 tbsp. olive oil

Instructions:

1. Ready your oven for baking at 350°F (175°C).
2. Pour the milk into the bowl and whisk in the eggs, salt, and pepper until well mixed.
3. Warm the olive oil in a skillet that can be used in the oven over medium heat.
4. Toss in the chopped veggies and sauté for 5-7 minutes, or until they start to soften.
5. After the veggies have been sautéed, pour the egg mixture over them.
6. Top the egg mixture with the shredded cheese.
7. After three or four minutes of cooking on the stove, the frittata should begin to solidify around the edges.
8. After a ten-to-fifteen-minute preheating, move the pan to the oven and continue baking until the frittata is set throughout and has a golden brown crust.
9. After a few minutes of cooling, take it out of the oven and cut it into serving pieces.
10. Savor every bite of that savory vegetable frittata!

Nutrition Information (per serving): Calories: ~250, Fat: ~18g, Carbohydrates: ~5g, Protein: ~15g

Chia Seed Pudding

Prep Time: 5 minutes (plus chilling time)

Cook Time: 0 minutes

Servings: 2

Ingredients:

- ¼ cup of chia seeds
- 1 cup of milk (dairy or plant-based)
- 1 tbsp. honey or maple syrup (optional)
- ½ **tsp** vanilla extract
- Toppings: fresh fruits, nuts, seeds, shredded coconut

Instructions:

1. Combine the chia seeds, milk, honey (or maple syrup, if using), and vanilla essence in a bowl and whisk to combine.
2. To avoid clumping, cover and chill for at least 2 hours, preferably overnight. Stir periodically.
3. Finish whisking the chia seed pudding just before

serving to ensure it reaches the thickness you like.

4. Transfer the pudding to individual serving dishes.
5. Add shredded coconut, fresh fruit, nuts, seeds, or whatever toppings you choose.
6. Enjoy your healthy chia seed pudding when served cold.

Nutrition Information (per serving): Calories: ~150, Fat: ~8g, Carbohydrates: ~15g, Protein: ~6g

<u>Egg Muffins</u>

Prep Time: 10 minutes

Cook Time: 20 minutes

Servings: 6

Ingredients:

- 6 eggs
- ¼ cup of milk (dairy or plant-based)
- 1 cup of chopped vegetables (such as bell peppers, onions, spinach)
- ½ cup of shredded cheese (such as cheddar, mozzarella)
- Salt and pepper to taste
- Optional add-ins: cooked bacon, diced ham, cooked sausage

Instructions:

1. Ready your oven for baking at 350°F (175°C). Melt some butter in a muffin pan or line it with paper liners.
2. Blend the eggs, milk, pepper, and salt in a bowl using a whisk.
3. Add the shredded cheese and diced veggies and mix well.
4. Pour the batter into the muffin tins, filling each one three quarters of the way to the top.
5. Sprinkle the optional toppings over each muffin cup of.
6. Before placing in the prepared oven, bake the egg muffins for 18 to 20 minutes, or until they set and have a little brown top.
7. After taking the egg muffins out of the muffin pan, let them cool for a while.
8. You may eat them warm or allow them to cool completely before keeping them in a sealed jar in the fridge for three or four days.
9. Whether you're having them for breakfast or a snack, these egg muffins will satisfy your hunger.

Nutrition Information (per serving, based on 1 muffin):

Calories: ~120, Fat: ~8g, Carbohydrates: ~3g, Protein: ~9g

Overnight Oats

Prep Time: 5 minutes (plus chilling time)

Cook Time: 0 minutes

Servings: 2

Ingredients:

- 1 cup of rolled oats
- 1 cup of milk (dairy or plant-based)
- 1 tbsp. chia seeds
- 1 tbsp. honey or maple syrup (optional)
- ½ **tsp** vanilla extract
- Toppings: sliced fruits, nuts, seeds, nut butter, yogurt

Instructions:

1. All of the ingredients— rolled oats, milk, chia seeds, honey, maple syrup, or vanilla extract—should be combined in a container or jar.
2. Make sure to mix everything well.
3. Put the lid on and chill for at least four hours, preferably overnight.
4. After the oats have slept, stir them again in the morning.
5. You may top it with sliced fruit, nuts, seeds, nut butter, or yogurt if you want.
6. Enjoy your tasty and healthy overnight oats cold.

Nutrition Information (per serving): Calories: ~250, Fat: ~6g, Carbohydrates: ~40g, Protein: ~8g

Greek Yogurt Parfait

Prep Time: 5 minutes

Cook Time: 0 minutes

Servings: 1

Ingredients:

- 1 cup of Greek yogurt (plain or flavored)
- ½ cup of granola
- ½ cup of mixed berries (such as strawberries, blueberries, raspberries)
- 1 tbsp. honey or maple syrup (optional)
- Optional add-ins: sliced bananas, nuts, seeds, shredded coconut

Instructions:

1. Arrange a serving dish or glass with granola, Greek yogurt, and a variety of berries.
2. Continue layering until the bowl or glass is full.
3. As an option, you may drizzle some maple syrup or honey on top.
4. Feel free to garnish it with sliced bananas, almonds, seeds, or shredded coconut, among other possible ingredients.
5. This healthy and delicious Greek yogurt parfait is ready to be enjoyed right away.

Nutrition Information (per serving): Calories: ~300, Fat: ~8g, Carbohydrates: ~45g, Protein: ~15g

Breakfast Burrito

Prep Time: 10 minutes

Cook Time: 10 minutes

Servings: 2

Ingredients:

- 4 large eggs
- ¼ cup of milk (dairy or plant-based)
- Salt and pepper to taste
- 1 tbsp. olive oil
- ½ cup of diced bell peppers
- ½ cup of diced onions
- ½ cup of diced tomatoes
- ½ cup of shredded cheese (such as cheddar or Monterey Jack)
- 2 large flour tortillas
- Optional toppings: salsa, avocado slices, sour cream

Instructions:

1. Pour the milk into the bowl and whisk in the eggs, salt, and pepper until well mixed.
2. In a pan, heat the olive oil over medium heat.
3. Simmer for three to four minutes, or until the onions and bell peppers are softened, after which add them to the skillet.
4. Toss in the diced tomatoes and continue cooking for another two minutes.
5. Scramble the eggs in a skillet after adding the egg mixture. Cook until done.
6. While the scrambled eggs are cooking, cover with grated cheese and set aside to melt.
7. To warm the flour tortillas, use a microwave or separate skillet.
8. Warm up several tortillas

and then divide the egg and cheese mixture among them.

9. Make burritos by rolling up the tortillas and folding in the edges.
10. Add salsa, avocado slices, and sour cream as toppings to the breakfast burritos if desired.
11. Your breakfast burritos are delicious and filling.

Nutrition Information:

Calories: ~400, Fat: ~20g, Carbohydrates: ~30g, Protein: ~20g

Cottage Cheese with Fruit

Prep Time: 5 minutes

Cook Time: 0 minutes

Servings: 1

Ingredients:

- ½ cup of cottage cheese
- ½ cup of mixed fruits (such as berries, sliced bananas, diced mango)
- 1 tbsp. honey or maple syrup (optional)
- Optional add-ins: nuts, seeds, shredded coconut

Instructions:

1. Spoon the cottage cheese into a serving dish.
2. Arrange a variety of fruits on top of the cottage cheese.
3. As an option, you may drizzle some maple syrup or honey on top.
4. Feel free to garnish it with shredded coconut, almonds, seeds, or whatever else you choose.
5. This easy and healthy cottage cheese with fruit is best enjoyed right away.

Nutrition Information (per serving): Calories: ~200, Fat: ~5g, Carbohydrates: ~25g, Protein: ~15g

Quinoa Breakfast Bowl

Prep Time: 5 minutes

Cook Time: 15 minutes

Servings: 2

Ingredients:

- 1 cup of cooked quinoa
- ½ cup of milk (dairy or plant-based)
- 1 tbsp. honey or maple syrup
- ½ **tsp** ground cinnamon
- ½ cup of mixed berries

(such as strawberries, blueberries, raspberries)
- ¼ cup of chopped nuts (such as almonds, walnuts)
- Optional add-ins: sliced bananas, diced mango, shredded coconut

Instructions:

1. Blend the cooked quinoa with the milk, honey (or maple syrup), and ground cinnamon in a saucepan.
2. Heat through, stirring periodically, over medium heat.
3. In separate dishes, distribute the quinoa mixture.
4. Various toppings, including chopped almonds, sliced bananas, mango, or shredded coconut, may be added on top, along with a combination of berries.
5. Enjoy this healthy and filling quinoa breakfast dish while it's still warm.

Nutrition Information (per serving, based on 2 servings):

Calories: ~300, Fat: ~10g, Carbohydrates: ~45g, Protein: ~10g

VEGETABLES AND SIDE DISHES

Zucchini Noodles (Zoodles)

Prep Time: 10 minutes

Cook Time: 5 minutes

Servings: 2

Ingredients:

- 2 medium zucchinis
- 1 tbsp. olive oil
- 2 cloves garlic, minced
- Salt and pepper to taste
- Optional toppings: grated Parmesan cheese, cherry tomatoes, fresh basil leaves

Instructions:

1. After you trim the ends of the zucchini, use a spiralizer to make noodles.
2. In a big skillet, heat the olive oil over medium heat.
3. Simmer for one or two minutes, or until aromatic, after which add the minced garlic to the pan.

4. After the oil has been infused with garlic, add the zucchini noodles and toss to coat.
5. Stir regularly while cooking the zucchini noodles for two to three minutes, or until they are barely cooked but retain a small crunch.
6. Adjust the seasoning with salt and pepper before serving the zucchini noodles.
7. Arrange the zucchini noodles on individual dishes and garnish with optional ingredients like cherry tomatoes, fresh basil, and grated Parmesan cheese.
8. Enjoy these tasty and healthy zucchini noodles (zoodles) right now!

Nutrition Information (per serving): Calories: ~60, Fat: ~4g, Carbohydrates: ~6g, Protein: ~2g

Steamed Broccoli with Lemon

Prep Time: 5 minutes

Cook Time: 5 minutes

Servings: 2

Ingredients:

- 2 cups of broccoli florets
- 1 tbsp. olive oil
- 1 tbsp. lemon juice
- Salt and pepper to taste
- Lemon zest (optional)

Instructions:

1. Add a steamer basket to a saucepan of water that is about an inch deep.
2. Heat the water in a saucepan over medium-high heat until it boils.
3. Place the broccoli florets in the steamer basket, cover, and cook for three to five minutes, or until the broccoli reaches a soft crispness while retaining its brilliant green color.
4. In the meantime, combine the lemon juice and olive oil in a small bowl and whisk to combine.
5. Move the cooked broccoli to a serving dish.
6. Pour the olive oil flavored with lemon over the broccoli that has been cooked.
7. Toss lightly to coat, then season with salt and pepper according to your taste.
8. If you like, you may top it off with lime zest.
9. Steamed broccoli with lemon, a healthy and easy

side dish, is ready to be enjoyed right away.

Nutrition Information (per serving):

Calories: ~50

Fat: ~4g

Carbohydrates: ~4g

Protein: ~2g

Roasted Brussels Sprouts

Prep Time: 10 minutes

Cook Time: 25 minutes

Servings: 4

Ingredients:

- 1 lb. Brussels sprouts, trimmed and halved
- 2 **tbsp.** olive oil
- 2 cloves garlic, minced
- Salt and pepper to taste
- Optional toppings: grated Parmesan cheese, balsamic glaze, chopped bacon

Instructions:

1. Line a baking sheet with foil or parchment paper and heat the oven to 400°F, or 200°C.
2. To coat the Brussels sprouts equally, toss them in a big basin with the olive oil, chopped garlic, salt, and pepper.
3. Once the baking sheet is ready, spread the Brussels sprouts out evenly.
4. To get soft and caramelized Brussels sprouts, roast them in a preheated oven for 20-25 minutes, stirring halfway through.
5. The roasted Brussels sprouts should be transferred to a serving plate after being removed from the oven.
6. If you like, you may top it with chopped bacon, balsamic glaze, or grated Parmesan cheese.
7. Enjoy your flavorful roasted Brussels sprouts right away by serving them hot.

Nutrition Information (per serving):

Calories: ~100

Fat: ~7g

Carbohydrates: ~9g

Protein: ~4g

Cauliflower Fried Rice

Prep Time: 15 minutes

Cook Time: 10 minutes

Servings: 4

Ingredients:

- 1 head cauliflower, riced (or 4 cups of pre-riced cauliflower)
- 2 **tbsp.** sesame oil (or olive oil)
- 2 cloves garlic, minced
- 1 small onion, diced
- 1 cup of mixed vegetables (such as diced carrots, peas, corn)
- 2 eggs, beaten
- 3 **tbsp.** soy sauce (or tamari for gluten-free)
- Optional toppings: sliced green onions, sesame seeds, Sirach sauce

Instructions:

1. If you don't have cauliflower that has been pre-riced, chop it into florets and pulse it until it looks like rice.
2. In a big wok or pan set over medium heat, warm the sesame oil.
3. Sauté the chopped onion and minced garlic for two or three minutes, or until aromatic.
4. After another three or four minutes, or until the veggies are soft, add the mixed vegetables to the pan.
5. Remove the veggies from the pan and pour the beaten eggs into the empty space. Cook the eggs by scrambling them.
6. Combine the cooked veggies and scrambled eggs in the skillet.
7. After the cauliflower has been riced, add the soy sauce and toss to mix.
8. Toss the cauliflower around every three to four minutes to cook it through and make sure it's soft.
9. Serve hot after removing from heat.
10. If you'd like, you may top it with chopped green onions, sesame seeds, or Sirach sauce.
11. Yummy and nutritious cauliflower fried rice—enjoy!

Nutrition Information (per serving):

Calories: ~150

Fat: ~8g

Carbohydrates: ~12g

Protein: ~8g

Grilled Asparagus

Prep Time: 5 minutes

Cook Time: 10 minutes

Servings: 4

Ingredients:

- 1 lb. asparagus spears, tough ends trimmed
- 2 **tbsp.** olive oil
- 2 cloves garlic, minced
- Salt and pepper to taste
- Optional toppings: grated Parmesan cheese, lemon zest, chopped almonds

Instructions:

1. Bring the grill up to a medium-high temperature.
2. Before serving, coat the asparagus spears well in a bowl with the olive oil, garlic, salt, and pepper.
3. Arrange the spears of asparagus in a single layer on the hot grill.
4. To get a little blackened and tender asparagus, grill it for around seven to eight minutes, flipping once.
5. After grilling, take the asparagus from the heat and place it on a dish for serving.
6. If you choose, you may garnish it with chopped almonds, lemon zest, or grated Parmesan cheese.
7. Enjoy your flavorful grilled asparagus right away by serving it hot.

Nutrition Information (per serving):

Calories: ~60

Fat: ~5g

Carbohydrates: ~4g

Protein: ~2g

Stuffed Bell Peppers

Prep Time: 20 minutes

Cook Time: 30 minutes

Servings: 4

Ingredients:

- 4 large bell peppers, any color
- 1 tbsp. olive oil
- 1 small onion, diced
- 2 cloves garlic, minced
- 1 lb. ground turkey or beef

- 1 cup of cooked rice (white or brown)
- 1 cup of diced tomatoes
- 1 **tsp** dried oregano
- 1 **tsp** dried basil
- Salt and pepper to taste
- 1 cup of shredded cheese (such as cheddar or mozzarella)
- Optional toppings: chopped fresh parsley, sour cream, salsa

Instructions:

1. Turn the oven on high heat (375°F, 190°C). The stuffed peppers will need a baking dish that can accommodate them, so grease it.
2. After halves the peppers, cut them in half lengthwise and scoop off the seeds and membranes. Put aside.
3. In a pan, heat the olive oil over medium heat.
4. Simmer for two or three minutes, or until the garlic and onion are softened, after which add the chopped onion to the pan.
5. Toss in some ground meat, such as turkey or beef, and brown it in a pan while breaking it up with a spoon.
6. After the rice is cooked, add the diced tomatoes, dried oregano and basil, salt, and pepper. Stir to combine. Heat thoroughly by cooking for another two or three minutes.
7. Evenly distribute the filling mixture into the bell peppers that have been hollowed out.
8. After you have the baking dish ready, put the filled peppers inside.
9. To make sure the peppers cook through, cover the baking dish with foil and bake it in a preheated oven for 25 to 30 minutes.
10. After stuffing the peppers, take off the foil and top with shredded cheese.
11. Make sure the cheese is melted and bubbling by returning the baking dish to the oven for another 5 minutes.
12. After taking the stuffed peppers out of the oven, give them a little time to cool down before you dig in.
13. Toppings like sour cream, salsa, chopped fresh parsley, and other condiments are optional.

14. These filled bell peppers are substantial and tasty; serve hot and savor!

Nutrition Information (per serving):

Calories: ~300

Fat: ~15g

Carbohydrates: ~20g

Protein: ~20g

Spinach and Mushroom Salad

Prep Time: 10 minutes

Cook Time: 0 minutes

Servings: 4

Ingredients:

- 6 cups of fresh spinach leaves
- 1 cup of sliced mushrooms
- ¼ cup of sliced red onions
- ¼ cup of crumbled feta cheese
- ¼ cup of chopped walnuts or almonds
- 2 **tbsp.** olive oil
- 2 **tbsp.** balsamic vinegar
- Salt and pepper to taste

Instructions:

1. Gently mix the fresh spinach leaves with the sliced mushrooms, red onions, crumbled feta cheese, chopped walnuts or almonds, and a big salad dish.
2. Dressing: In a small bowl, mix together balsamic vinegar and olive oil.
3. Slightly coat the salad with the dressing by pouring it over it and tossing slightly.
4. Taste and add salt and pepper as needed.
5. Quickly prepare and enjoy this revitalizing salad of spinach and mushrooms.

Nutrition Information (per serving):

Calories: ~150

Fat: ~12g

Carbohydrates: ~8g

Protein: ~5g

Garlic Parmesan Green Beans

Prep Time: 10 minutes

Cook Time: 10 minutes

Servings: 4

Ingredients:

- 1 lb. green beans, trimmed
- 2 **tbsp.** olive oil
- 2 cloves garlic, minced
- ¼ cup of grated Parmesan cheese
- Salt and pepper to taste
- Lemon wedges for serving (optional)

Instructions:

1. Heat up a big saucepan of water until it boils. Once the green beans are brilliant green and somewhat crunchy, add them to the pan and cook for another two or three minutes.
2. Once the green beans have drained, drop them into a basin of cold water to halt cooking. Pat dry with paper towels and drain one more.
3. With the heat set to medium, warm the olive oil in a big skillet. Sauté the minced garlic for a minute or two, until it begins to release its aroma.
4. Coat the blanched green beans uniformly with the garlic-infused oil by adding them to the pan and tossing.
5. To make the green beans soft, cook for three to four minutes, stirring once or twice.
6. After you toss the green beans, top them with the shredded Parmesan cheese.
7. Taste and add salt and pepper as needed.
8. Put the green beans with garlic and parmesan sauce on a serving dish after taking them from the stove.
9. If preferred, serve hot and garnish with lemon wedges.
10. Garlic parmesan green beans are a healthy and delicious side dish.

Nutrition Information (per serving):

Calories: ~100

Fat: ~7g

Carbohydrates: ~7g

Protein: ~3g

Ratatouille

Prep Time: 20 minutes

Cook Time: 40 minutes

Servings: 4

Ingredients:

- 1 eggplant, diced
- 2 zucchinis, diced
- 1 yellow bell pepper, diced
- 1 red bell pepper, diced
- 1 onion, diced
- 2 cloves garlic, minced
- 2 cups of diced tomatoes (fresh or canned)
- 2 **tbsp.** tomato paste
- 2 **tbsp.** olive oil
- 1 **tsp** dried thyme
- 1 **tsp** dried oregano
- Salt and pepper to taste
- Fresh basil leaves for garnish (optional)

Instructions:

1. Toss the olive oil into a big Dutch oven or pan and set it over medium heat.
2. Sauté the minced garlic and chopped onion for three to four minutes, or until the onions are tender.
3. Sauté the bell peppers, eggplant, and zucchini in a pan with some sliced onion. The veggies will begin to soften after about 7 to 10 minutes of cooking, stirring them periodically.
4. Toss in the tomato paste, chopped tomatoes, dried oregano and thyme, salt, and pepper.
5. Simmer, covered, for 20–25 minutes (stirring periodically), or until veggies are soft and flavors combine.
6. Reevaluate the seasoning according to your taste.
7. Take off the heat and let the ratatouille to cool for a little before you serve it.
8. Optional: top with a few fresh basil leaves for garnish.
9. As an entree or side dish, serve warm.
10. I hope you like this hearty ratatouille dish.

Nutrition Information (per serving):

Calories: ~150

Fat: ~7g

Carbohydrates: ~20g

Protein: ~4g

Cucumber Tomato Salad

Prep Time: 10 minutes

Cook Time: 0 minutes

Servings: 4

Ingredients:

- 2 large cucumbers, diced
- 2 cups of cherry tomatoes, halved
- ¼ cup of red onion, thinly sliced
- 2 **tbsp.** olive oil
- 1 tbsp. red wine vinegar
- 1 **tsp** Dijon mustard
- 1 tbsp. chopped fresh parsley
- Salt and pepper to taste
- Crumbled feta cheese for garnish (optional)

Instructions:

1. Mix the cherry tomatoes, chopped cucumbers, and sliced red onion in a big salad bowl.
2. The dressing is made by whisking togcthcr olive oil, red wine vinegar, Dijon mustard, chopped fresh parsley, salt, and pepper in a small bowl.
3. Toss the cucumber-tomato combination carefully to coat it with the dressing.
4. Reevaluate the seasoning according to your taste.
5. If you want, you may top it with crumbled feta cheese.
6. Keep in the fridge until serving time or serve right away.
7. Curious about cucumber tomato salad? Try this colorful and pleasant recipe!

Nutrition Information (per serving):

Calories: ~90

Fat: ~7g

Carbohydrates: ~7g

Protein: ~2g

Butternut Squash Soup

Prep Time: 15 minutes

Cook Time: 45 minutes

Servings: 6

Ingredients:

- 1 medium butternut squash, peeled, seeded, and diced
- 1 onion, diced
- 2 carrots, diced
- 2 stalks celery, diced
- 2 cloves garlic, minced
- 4 cups of vegetable broth
- 1 **tsp** dried thyme
- ½ **tsp** ground cinnamon
- Salt and pepper to taste
- 2 **tbsp.** olive oil
- Optional toppings: roasted pumpkin seeds, drizzle of cream, chopped fresh herbs

Instructions:

1. Turn the oven on high heat (400°F, 200°C).
2. Bake the butternut squash, onion, carrots, and celery chopped. Olive oil, salt, and pepper should be drizzled over top. Put in the coat.
3. To get soft and caramelized veggies, roast them in a preheated oven for 25 to 30 minutes.
4. Warm up some olive oil in a big saucepan over medium heat. Cook for 1 minute, or until aromatic, then add minced garlic.
5. Incorporate the roasted veggies into the sauce. After adding the ground cinnamon and dried thyme, pour in the vegetable broth. Simmer for a few minutes.
6. Let the flavors combine by simmering for around fifteen minutes.
7. To get a smooth purée, mix the soup using an immersion blender. You might also use a blender to puree the soup in portions. Handle hot liquids with caution when combining.
8. Toss in some salt and pepper to season the soup.
9. Warm the dish before serving; if preferred, top with toasted pumpkin seeds, a splash of cream, and chopped fresh herbs.
10. Butternut squash soup is a hearty and satisfying dish; savor it.

Nutrition Information (per serving):

Calories: ~150

Fat: ~5g

Carbohydrates: ~25g

Protein: ~3g

<u>Roasted Root Vegetables</u>

Prep Time: 15 minutes

Cook Time: 40 minutes

Servings: 6

Ingredients:

- 2 carrots, peeled and cut into chunks
- 2 parsnips, peeled and cut into chunks
- 2 beets, peeled and cut into chunks
- 1 sweet potato, peeled and cut into chunks
- 1 red onion, peeled and cut into wedges

- 2 **tbsp.** olive oil
- 2 cloves garlic, minced
- 1 **tsp** dried thyme
- Salt and pepper to taste
- Optional toppings: chopped fresh parsley, crumbled feta cheese, balsamic glaze

Instructions:

1. Turn the oven on high heat (400°F, 200°C).
2. Roast the red onion, sweet potato, beets, parsnips, and carrots in a large baking dish.
3. In a bowl, combine the chopped garlic, dried thyme, salt, and pepper with the olive oil. Toss the veggies to coat. Whisk to combine.
4. On the baking sheet, arrange the veggies in a single layer.
5. To produce soft and caramelized veggies, roast them in a preheated oven for 35 to 40 minutes, stirring once halfway through.
6. After the root vegetables have roasted, take them out of the oven and place them on a serving platter.
7. Add toppings like crumbled feta cheese, minced fresh parsley, or a splash of balsamic glaze if you choose.
8. The roasted root vegetables are beautiful and full of flavor; serve hot and savor!

Nutrition Information (per serving):

Calories: ~150

Fat: ~5g

Carbohydrates: ~25g

Protein: ~3g

Kale Chips

Prep Time: 10 minutes

Cook Time: 15 minutes

Servings: 4

Ingredients:

- 1 bunch kale, stems removed and torn into bite-sized pieces
- 1 tbsp. olive oil
- Salt to taste
- Optional seasonings: garlic powder, onion powder, paprika, grated Parmesan cheese

Instructions:

1. The oven should be preheated to 300°F, or 150°C. Gather parchment paper and set it aside.

2. Coat the kale pieces equally with olive oil by tossing them in a big basin.
3. Arrange the kale in a single layer on the baking sheet that has been prepared.
4. Season with salt and anything else you want.
5. Toss the kale halfway through baking in a preheated oven for 10 to 15 minutes, or until it becomes crispy without being burned.
6. Take it out of the oven and give it a little time to cool down before you dig in.
7. Munch on some healthy kale chips for a crisp snack or side.

Nutrition Information (per serving):

Calories: ~50

Fat: ~3g

Carbohydrates: ~5g

Protein: ~2g

Sweet Potato Fries

Prep Time: 15 minutes

Cook Time: 25 minutes

Servings: 4

Ingredients:

- 2 large sweet potatoes, peeled and cut into fries
- 2 **tbsp.** olive oil
- 1 **tsp** paprika
- ½ **tsp** garlic powder
- Salt and pepper to taste

Instructions:

1. Set the oven temperature to 425°F, or 220°C. Gather parchment paper and set it aside.
2. Combine the sweet potato fries in a big bowl and sprinkle them equally with olive oil, paprika, garlic powder, salt, and pepper.
3. Once the baking sheet is ready, spread the sweet potato fries out evenly.
4. Fries need to be cooked in a preheated oven for 20 to 25 minutes, turning once halfway through, or until they become crispy and golden.
5. Take it out of the oven and give it a little time to cool down before you dig in.
6. Crispy sweet potato fries dipped in your preferred sauce are sure to satisfy your cravings.

Nutrition Information (per serving):

Calories: ~150

Fat: ~7g

Carbohydrates: ~20g

Protein: ~2g

<u>Balsamic Glazed Carrots</u>

Prep Time: 10 minutes

Cook Time: 20 minutes

Servings: 4

Ingredients:

- 1 lb. carrots, peeled and sliced into sticks
- 2 **tbsp.** olive oil
- 2 **tbsp.** balsamic vinegar
- 1 tbsp. honey or maple syrup
- Salt and pepper to taste
- Optional garnish: chopped fresh parsley

Instructions:

1. Turn the oven on high heat (400°F, 200°C). Gather parchment paper and set it aside.
2. Whisk together the balsamic vinegar, honey or maple syrup, salt, and pepper in a bowl. Coat the carrot sticks equally.
3. Arrange the carrots in a single layer on the baking sheet that has been preheated.
4. To get soft and caramelized carrots, bake in a preheated oven for 15 to 20 minutes, stirring halfway through.
5. Take it out of the oven and give it a little time to cool down before you dig in.
6. If you want, you may top it off with some chopped fresh parsley.
7. As a delectable accompaniment, savor these carrots coated in a sweet and tart balsamic glaze.

Nutrition Information (per serving):

Calories: ~100

Fat: ~5g

Carbohydrates: ~15g

Protein: ~1g

SOUP

Skinny Taco Soup

Prep Time: 15 minutes

Cook Time: 25 minutes

Servings: 6

Ingredients:

- 1 lb. lean ground turkey
- 1 onion, chopped
- 1 bell pepper, diced
- 1 can (15 oz.) black beans, drained and rinsed
- 1 can (15 oz.) kidney beans, drained and rinsed
- 1 can (15 oz.) corn, drained
- 1 can (15 oz.) diced tomatoes
- 1 packet low-sodium taco seasoning
- 4 cups of low-sodium chicken broth
- Optional toppings: shredded cheese, diced avocado, Greek yogurt, cilantro

Instructions:

1. Ground turkey should be brown in a big saucepan over medium heat.
2. After the onion and bell pepper are chopped, add them to the saucepan and simmer until they are soft.
3. Before adding chicken stock, black beans, kidney beans, corn, chopped tomatoes, and taco spice, stir everything together.
4. Simmer the soup for 20 minutes after bringing it to a boil.
5. Garnish with chopped avocado, Greek yogurt, cilantro, and shredded cheese if desired. Serve hot.

Nutrition Information (per serving):

Calories: 280

Total Fat: 5g

Cholesterol: 40mg

Sodium: 680mg

Total Carbohydrates: 37g

Dietary Fiber: 9g

Sugars: 6g

Protein: 24g

Vegetable Soup

Prep Time: 15 minutes

Cook Time: 30 minutes

Servings: 8

Ingredients:

- 1 tbsp. olive oil
- 1 onion, chopped
- 2 carrots, sliced

- 2 celery stalks, sliced
- 2 cloves garlic, minced
- 1 can (14 oz.) diced tomatoes
- 6 cups of vegetable broth
- 2 cups of chopped vegetables (e.g., zucchini, bell peppers, green beans)
- 1 **tsp** dried thyme
- Salt and pepper to taste
- Fresh parsley for garnish (optional)

Instructions:

1. Olive oil should be heated in a big saucepan over medium heat. Slicing carrots and celery and adding chopped onion completes the recipe. After around 5 minutes of cooking, the veggies should be tender.
2. For another minute, or until aromatic, add the minced garlic.
3. Add the veggie broth and diced tomatoes. Simmer until it begins to boil.
4. Chop the veggies and add the dried thyme after the water boils. Simmer, covered, for 20 to 25 minutes, or until veggies are soft, or until heat is reduced to low.
5. Taste and add salt and pepper as needed.
6. Hot, with fresh parsley as a garnish, if desired.

Nutrition Information (per serving):

Calories: 110

Total Fat: 3g

Cholesterol: 0mg

Sodium: 650mg

Total Carbohydrates: 19g

Dietary Fiber: 5g

Sugars: 7g

Protein: 3g

<u>**Chicken Tortilla Soup**</u>

Prep Time: 15 minutes

Cook Time: 25 minutes

Servings: 6

Ingredients:

- 1 tbsp. olive oil
- 1 onion, chopped
- 2 cloves garlic, minced
- 1 jalapeño, seeded and diced
- 1 **tsp** ground cumin
- 1 **tsp** chili powder
- 1 can (14.5 oz.) diced tomatoes

- 1 can (15 oz.) black beans, drained and rinsed
- 1 can (15 oz.) corn, drained
- 4 cups of low-sodium chicken broth
- 2 cups of shredded cooked chicken breast
- Salt and pepper to taste
- Tortilla chips, avocado, shredded cheese, lime wedges for serving

Instructions:

1. Olive oil should be heated in a big saucepan over medium heat. Sauté the chopped onion for about 5 minutes, or until it softens.
2. After 2 more minutes, add the minced garlic and diced jalapeño.
3. Cook, stirring occasionally, for 1 minute, or until aromatic, adding ground cumin and chili powder.
4. Throw in some corn, black beans, chopped tomatoes, and chicken broth. Simmer for a few minutes.
5. Substitute shredded chicken breast once it has simmered. Add another 15 minutes of cooking time to the soup.
6. Taste and add salt and pepper as needed.
7. Top with avocado, shredded cheese, lime wedges, tortilla chips, and serve hot.

Nutrition Information (per serving):

Calories: 280

Total Fat: 8g

Cholesterol: 35mg

Sodium: 550mg

Total Carbohydrates: 31g

Dietary Fiber: 8g

Sugars: 5g

Protein: 23g

Italian Wedding Soup

Prep Time: 20 minutes

Cook Time: 30 minutes

Servings: 6

Ingredients:

- 1 tbsp. olive oil
- 1 onion, finely chopped
- 2 carrots, diced
- 2 celery stalks, diced
- 2 cloves garlic, minced
- 8 cups of low-sodium chicken broth
- 1 cup of small pasta (such as acini di pepe or orzo)

- 1 lb. lean ground turkey or chicken
- 1 egg, beaten
- ¼ cup of grated Parmesan cheese
- 2 **tbsp.** chopped fresh parsley
- Salt and pepper to taste
- Fresh spinach leaves
- Lemon wedges for serving (optional)

Instructions:

1. Warm the olive oil in a big saucepan over medium heat. Toss in some diced carrots, celery, and onion. After around 5 minutes of cooking, the veggies should be tender.
2. For a minute, or until aromatic, add the minced garlic.
3. Add the chicken broth and reduce heat to low.
4. Besides that, in a mixing bowl, mix together the ground meat (chicken or turkey), beaten egg, grated Parmesan cheese, chopped parsley, salt, and pepper. Shape into little meatballs after thoroughly mixing.
5. Toss in the meatballs and little spaghetti once the stock has simmered. Once the meatballs are cooked and the spaghetti is soft, around 10 to 12 minutes should be enough cooking time.
6. Cook, stirring occasionally, until the fresh spinach wilts.
7. Season with salt and pepper according to your preference.
8. Warm the soup before serving; garnish with lemon slices, if desired.

Nutrition Information (per serving):

Calories: 320

Total Fat: 10g

Cholesterol: 70mg

Sodium: 660mg

Total Carbohydrates: 28g

Dietary Fiber: 3g

Sugars: 5g

Protein: 27g

Minestrone Soup

Prep Time: 15 minutes

Cook Time: 30 minutes

Servings: 8

Ingredients:

- 2 **tbsp.** olive oil
- 1 onion, chopped
- 2 carrots, diced
- 2 celery stalks, diced
- 3 cloves garlic, minced
- 1 can (14.5 oz.) diced tomatoes
- 6 cups of vegetable broth
- 1 can (15 oz.) kidney beans, drained and rinsed
- 1 can (15 oz.) cannellini beans, drained and rinsed
- 1 cup of small pasta
- 1 **tsp** dried oregano
- 1 **tsp** dried basil
- Salt and pepper to taste
- Freshly grated Parmesan cheese for serving
- Fresh basil leaves for garnish (optional)

Instructions:

1. Olive oil should be heated in a big saucepan over medium heat. Toss in some diced carrots, celery, and onion. After around 5 minutes of cooking, the veggies should be tender.
2. For a minute, or until aromatic, add the minced garlic.
3. Add the veggie broth and diced tomatoes. Simmer for a few minutes.
4. Once the sauce has simmered, stir in the kidney beans, cannellini beans, tiny pasta, dry oregano, and dried basil that have been drained and washed. Once the pasta is soft, cook it for another 10 to 12 minutes.
5. Taste and add salt and pepper as needed.
6. When ready to serve, top with grated Parmesan and basil leaves, if preferred.

Nutrition Information (per serving):

Calories: 280

Total Fat: 5g

Cholesterol: 0mg

Sodium: 800mg

Total Carbohydrates: 48g

Dietary Fiber: 10g

Sugars: 7g

Protein: 12g

Lentil Soup

Prep Time: 10 minutes

Cook Time: 40 minutes

Servings: 6

Ingredients:

- 1 tbsp. olive oil
- 1 onion, chopped
- 2 carrots, diced
- 2 celery stalks, diced
- 3 cloves garlic, minced
- 1 cup of dried lentils, rinsed and drained
- 6 cups of vegetable broth
- 1 can (14.5 oz.) diced tomatoes
- 1 **tsp** ground cumin
- 1 **tsp** paprika
- Salt and pepper to taste
- Fresh parsley for garnish (optional)

Instructions:

1. In a big saucepan, warm the olive oil over medium heat. Toss in some diced carrots, celery, and onion. After around 5 minutes of cooking, the veggies should be tender.
2. For a minute, or until aromatic, add the minced garlic.
3. Add the vegetable broth, diced tomatoes, dry lentils, ground cumin, and paprika, and stir to combine.
4. Simmer, covered, for 30–35 minutes, or until lentils are soft, after bringing to a boil.
5. Add salt and pepper according to your preference.
6. Garnish with fresh parsley if desired and serve hot.

Nutrition Information (per serving):

Calories: 220

Total Fat: 3g

Cholesterol: 0mg

Sodium: 750mg

Total Carbohydrates: 37g

Dietary Fiber: 15g

Sugars: 6g

Protein: 13g

Creamy Cauliflower Soup

Prep Time: 10 minutes

Cook Time: 30 minutes

Servings: 4

Ingredients:

- 1 head cauliflower, chopped into florets
- 1 onion, chopped
- 2 cloves garlic, minced
- 2 **tbsp.** olive oil
- 4 cups of vegetable broth

- ½ cup of heavy cream
- Salt and pepper to taste
- Fresh chives or parsley for garnish (optional)

Instructions:

1. Slowly bring olive oil to a simmer in a big saucepan. Cook, stirring occasionally, for about 5 minutes, until the garlic and onion are softened.
2. After the first 5 minutes, add the chopped cauliflower florets and continue cooking.
3. To make the cauliflower soft, add the vegetable broth, bring to a boil, then decrease heat and simmer for 15 to 20 minutes.
4. Puree the soup until its smooth either using an immersion blender or by transferring it to a blender.
5. Heavy cream should be stirred in after seasoning with salt and pepper.
6. Add 5 more minutes of cooking time to heat everything thoroughly.
7. Top with chopped parsley or fresh chives and serve hot.

Nutrition Information (per serving):

Calories: 210

Total Fat: 17g

Cholesterol: 30mg

Sodium: 830mg

Total Carbohydrates: 11g

Dietary Fiber: 4g

Sugars: 5g

Protein: 4g

Thai Curry Soup

Prep Time: 15 minutes

Cook Time: 25 minutes

Servings: 4

Ingredients:

- 1 tbsp. vegetable oil
- 1 onion, chopped
- 2 cloves garlic, minced
- 1 tbsp. Thai red curry paste
- 1 can (14 oz.) coconut milk
- 4 cups of chicken or vegetable broth
- 2 cups of chopped mixed vegetables (such as bell peppers, broccoli, and carrots)
- 1 cup of cooked chicken breast, shredded (optional)
- 1 tbsp. fish sauce (optional)
- Juice of 1 lime

- Salt and pepper to taste
- Fresh cilantro for garnish (optional)
- Cooked rice or noodles for serving

Instructions:

1. With a big saucepan set over medium heat, warm the vegetable oil. Cook, stirring occasionally, for about 5 minutes, until the garlic and onion are softened.
2. After a minute of cooking, add the Thai red curry paste and stir until it releases its aroma.
3. Add coconut milk and broth, whether it's chicken or vegetables. Simmer for a few minutes.
4. Before serving, top with cooked chicken breast and chopped mixed veggies. After ten to fifteen minutes of cooking, the veggies should be soft.
5. Toss in the lime juice and fish sauce, if using. Add salt and pepper according to your preference.
6. With cooked rice or noodles, top with chopped fresh cilantro and serve hot.

Nutrition Information (per serving):

Calories: 280

Total Fat: 21g

Cholesterol: 15mg

Sodium: 950mg

Total Carbohydrates: 15g

Dietary Fiber: 3g

Sugars: 5g

Protein: 9g

Turkey Chili

Prep Time: 15 minutes

Cook Time: 45 minutes

Servings: 6

Ingredients:

- 1 tbsp. olive oil
- 1 onion, chopped
- 2 cloves garlic, minced
- 1 bell pepper, diced
- 1 lb. ground turkey
- 2 cans (14.5 oz. each) diced tomatoes
- 1 can (15 oz.) kidney beans, drained and rinsed
- 1 can (15 oz.) black beans, drained and rinsed
- 1 cup of corn kernels (fresh, frozen, or canned)

- 2 **tbsp.** chili powder
- 1 **tsp** ground cumin
- 1 **tsp** paprika
- Salt and pepper to taste
- Optional toppings: shredded cheese, diced avocado, chopped cilantro, sour cream

Instructions:

1. In a big saucepan, warm the olive oil over medium heat. Incorporate diced bell pepper, minced garlic, and chopped onion. After around 5 minutes of cooking, the veggies should be tender.
2. Brown the ground turkey in a skillet while breaking it up with a spoon.
3. Toss in chopped tomatoes and their juices, kidney beans, black beans, corn kernels, paprika, chili powder, powdered cumin, and rinsed and drained black beans.
4. Add salt and pepper according to your preference.
5. After the chili comes to a boil, lower the heat to low and simmer, stirring regularly, for 30 to 40 minutes.
6. Top with sour cream, chopped cilantro, sliced

avocado, and shredded cheese if desired. Serve hot.

Nutrition Information (per serving):

Calories: 320

Total Fat: 8g

Cholesterol: 45mg

Sodium: 800mg

Total Carbohydrates: 38g

Dietary Fiber: 11g

Sugars: 7g

Protein: 27g

Butternut Squash Soup

Prep Time: 15 minutes

Cook Time: 45 minutes

Servings: 6

Ingredients:

- 1 tbsp. olive oil
- 1 onion, chopped
- 2 cloves garlic, minced
- 1 medium butternut squash, peeled, seeded, and diced
- 2 carrots, peeled and chopped
- 4 cups of vegetable or chicken broth
- 1 **tsp** ground cinnamon

- ½ **tsp** ground nutmeg
- Salt and pepper to taste
- ½ cup of heavy cream (optional)
- Toasted pumpkin seeds for garnish (optional)

Instructions:

1. In a big saucepan, warm the olive oil over medium heat. Cook, stirring occasionally, for about 5 minutes, until the garlic and onion are softened.
2. Toss in some sliced carrots and cubed butternut squash. Add 5 more minutes of cooking time.
3. Ground nutmeg, cinnamon, and vegetable or chicken broth should be added. Simmer for a few minutes.
4. Simmer the soup for twenty-five to thirty minutes, or until the carrots and butternut squash are soft.
5. Puree the soup until it's smooth either using an immersion blender or by transferring it to a blender.
6. To make the soup creamier, if desired, whisk in heavy cream. Add salt and pepper according to your preference.
7. Warm the dish before serving; toasted pumpkin seeds are an optional garnish.

Nutrition Information (per serving):

Calories: 180

Total Fat: 6g

Cholesterol: 20mg

Sodium: 680mg

Total Carbohydrates: 30g

Dietary Fiber: 5g

Sugars: 8g

Protein: 4g

<u>Zucchini Soup</u>

Prep Time: 10 minutes

Cook Time: 25 minutes

Servings: 4

Ingredients:

- 2 **tbsp.** olive oil
- 1 onion, chopped
- 2 cloves garlic, minced
- 4 medium zucchinis, chopped
- 4 cups of vegetable broth
- Salt and pepper to taste

- ¼ cup of grated Parmesan cheese (optional)
- Fresh parsley or basil for garnish (optional)

Instructions:

1. In a big saucepan, warm the olive oil over medium heat. Cook, stirring occasionally, for about 5 minutes, until the garlic and onion are softened.
2. Cook for a further 5 minutes after adding the chopped zucchini to the saucepan.
3. Once the zucchinis are soft, add the vegetable broth and boil for 15 minutes.
4. Puree the soup until it's smooth either using an immersion blender or by transferring it to a blender.
5. Add salt and pepper according to your preference.
6. Warm the dish before serving; if desired, top with grated Parmesan and chopped fresh basil or parsley.

Nutrition Information (per serving, without Parmesan cheese):

Calories: 100

Total Fat: 7g

Cholesterol: 0mg

Sodium: 650mg

Total Carbohydrates: 8g

Dietary Fiber: 2g

Sugars: 4g

Protein: 2g

Tomato Basil Soup

Prep Time: 10 minutes

Cook Time: 30 minutes

Servings: 4

Ingredients:

- 2 **tbsp.** olive oil
- 1 onion, chopped
- 2 cloves garlic, minced
- 2 cans (14.5 oz. each) diced tomatoes
- 1 can (14.5 oz.) tomato sauce
- 2 cups of vegetable broth
- ¼ cup of chopped fresh basil leaves
- Salt and pepper to taste
- ¼ cup of heavy cream (optional)
- Fresh basil leaves for garnish (optional)

Instructions:

1. In a big saucepan, warm the olive oil over medium heat. Cook, stirring occasionally, for about 5 minutes, until the garlic and onion are softened.
2. Toss in some chopped basil leaves, some tomato sauce, some diced tomatoes (together with their juices), and some veggie broth. Simmer for a few minutes.
3. Simmer, stirring periodically, for 20 minutes to allow the soup to thicken.
4. Puree the soup until its smooth either using an immersion blender or by transferring it to a blender.
5. To make the soup creamier, if desired, whisk in heavy cream. Add salt and pepper according to your preference.
6. Warm the dish before serving; fresh basil leaves are an optional garnish.

Nutrition Information (per serving, without heavy cream):

Calories: 140

Total Fat: 7g

Cholesterol: 0mg

Sodium: 780mg

Total Carbohydrates: 18g

Dietary Fiber: 4g

Sugars: 11g

Protein: 3g

SALADS

Grilled Chicken Caesar Salad

Prep Time: 15 minutes

Cook Time: 15 minutes

Servings: 4

Ingredients:

- 2 boneless, skinless chicken breasts
- 1 tbsp. olive oil
- Salt and pepper to taste
- 1 head romaine lettuce, chopped
- ½ cup of Caesar dressing

- ¼ cup of grated Parmesan cheese
- Croutons (optional)

Instructions:

1. Grill over medium-high heat until hot.
2. After seasoning the chicken breasts with salt and pepper, rub them with olive oil.
3. To cook the chicken thoroughly, grill it for around 6 to 7 minutes on each side. After taking it from the grill, let it a few minutes to rest before cutting.
4. Chopped romaine lettuce and Caesar dressing should be mixed in a big basin. Mix until all parts are covered.
5. On each dish, distribute the dressed lettuce.
6. Pile grilled chicken slices on top of each serving dish.
7. If you like, you may top it with croutons and grated Parmesan cheese.
8. Enjoy right away after serving!

Nutrition Information:

Calories: 350 per serving

Protein: 25g

Fat: 22g

Carbohydrates: 12g

Fiber: 4g

Quinoa and Black Bean Salad

Prep Time: 20 minutes

Cook Time: 15 minutes (for quinoa)

Servings: 6

Ingredients:

- 1 cup of quinoa, rinsed
- 2 cups of water or vegetable broth
- 1 can (15 oz.) black beans, drained and rinsed
- 1 red bell pepper, diced
- ½ cup of diced red onion
- ¼ cup of chopped fresh cilantro
- Juice of 2 limes
- 2 **tbsp.** olive oil
- 1 **tsp** ground cumin
- Salt and pepper to taste
- Optional toppings: avocado, cherry tomatoes, diced cucumber

Instructions:

1. Boil some water or veggie broth in a medium pot. Before the quinoa is cooked

and the water is absorbed, bring the pot to a low simmer, cover, and decrease heat to low. Simmer for 15 minutes. Take off the stove and let it cool.
2. The cooked quinoa, black beans, bell pepper, red onion, and cilantro should all be mixed together in a generous dish.
3. Stir the lime juice, olive oil, cumin powder, salt, and pepper in a small bowl.
4. Coat the quinoa mixture evenly by pouring the dressing over it and tossing.
5. If needed, taste and make adjustments to the seasoning.
6. If you want to add toppings, you may do so before serving, either cold or room temperature.
7. Savor it as an accompaniment or a lighter entrée!

Nutrition Information:

Calories: 250 per serving

Protein: 9g

Fat: 7g

Carbohydrates: 38g

Fiber: 8g

Mediterranean Chickpea Salad

Prep Time: 15 minutes

Cook Time: 0 minutes

Servings: 4

Ingredients:

- 2 cans (15 oz. each) chickpeas, drained and rinsed
- 1 cucumber, diced
- 1 bell pepper, diced
- 1 pint cherry tomatoes, halved
- ½ red onion, thinly sliced
- ¼ cup of Kalamata olives, pitted and halved
- ¼ cup of crumbled feta cheese
- ¼ cup of chopped fresh parsley
- ¼ cup of extra virgin olive oil
- 2 **tbsp.** red wine vinegar
- 1 **tsp** dried oregano
- Salt and pepper to taste

Instructions:

1. Throw everything into a big bowl and stir in the chickpeas, bell pepper, cucumber, cherry tomatoes,

and red onion, halved Kalamata olives, crumbled feta cheese, and chopped fresh parsley.

2. The dressing is made by whisking together red wine vinegar, dried oregano, salt, pepper, extra virgin olive oil, and a small bowl.
3. After combining the salad components, pour the dressing over them and mix well.
4. To make the tastes more harmonious, serve right away or let sit in the fridge for at least one or two hours.

Nutrition Information (per serving):

Calories: 320

Total Fat: 15g

Cholesterol: 5mg

Sodium: 480mg

Total Carbohydrates: 38g

Dietary Fiber: 10g

Sugars: 7g

Protein: 12g

Asian Sesame Chicken Salad

Prep Time: 20 minutes

Cook Time: 15 minutes

Servings: 4

Ingredients:

- 2 boneless, skinless chicken breasts
- Salt and pepper to taste
- 6 cups of mixed salad greens (e.g., lettuce, spinach, arugula)
- 1 carrot, julienned
- 1 cucumber, julienned
- 1 bell pepper, thinly sliced
- ¼ cup of chopped cilantro
- ¼ cup of chopped green onions
- ¼ cup of sliced almonds, toasted
- ¼ cup of crispy chow Mein noodles (optional)
- Sesame seeds for garnish (optional)
- For the Dressing:
- 2 **tbsp.** soy sauce
- 1 tbsp. rice vinegar
- 1 tbsp. sesame oil
- 1 tbsp. honey
- 1 clove garlic, minced
- 1 **tsp** grated ginger
- 1 tbsp. water

Instructions:

1. Lb. or season the chicken breasts with pepper and salt. Cook for about 6 to 7 minutes on each side whether grilled or pan-seared. After a little cooling, cut into strips.
2. Toss together the salad greens, cucumber, carrot, bell pepper, cilantro, green onions, toasted almonds, and crispy chow mein noodles (if using) in a big bowl.
3. To prepare the dressing, combine the following ingredients in a small bowl: rice vinegar, water, honey, sesame oil, garlic powder, ginger root, and soy sauce. Whisk until well combined.
4. Toss the salad dish with the cut chicken.
5. Toss the salad to cover it evenly with the dressing after you drizzle it over it.
6. Sesame seeds may be used as a garnish if preferred.
7. Make sure to serve right away.

Nutrition Information (per serving):

Calories: 280

Total Fat: 12g

Cholesterol: 40mg

Sodium: 580mg

Total Carbohydrates: 19g

Dietary Fiber: 4g

Sugars: 10g

Caprese Salad with Balsamic Glaze

Prep Time: 10 minutes

Cook Time: 0 minutes

Servings: 4

Ingredients:

- 2 large tomatoes, sliced
- 1 ball fresh mozzarella cheese, sliced
- Fresh basil leaves
- Salt and pepper to taste
- Balsamic glaze (store-bought or homemade)

Instructions:

1. Put the mozzarella cheese and tomatoes on a serving plate in alternate rows.
2. Sandwich the tomato and mozzarella slices with fresh basil leaves tucked in.
3. Add salt and pepper according to your preference.

4. Pour balsamic glaze over the top.
5. Quickly serve as a revitalizing appetizer or accompaniment.

Nutrition Information (per serving):

Calories: 160

Total Fat: 10g

Cholesterol: 30mg

Sodium: 230mg

Total Carbohydrates: 6g

Dietary Fiber: 1g

Sugars: 4g

Protein: 11g

<u>Southwest Shrimp Salad</u>

Prep Time: 15 minutes

Cook Time: 5 minutes

Servings: 4

Ingredients:

- 1 lb. large shrimp, peeled and deveined
- 1 tbsp. olive oil
- 1 **tsp** chili powder
- 1 **tsp** cumin
- ½ **tsp** garlic powder
- Salt and pepper to taste
- 6 cups of mixed salad greens
- 1 cup of cherry tomatoes, halved
- ½ cup of corn kernels (fresh, canned, or frozen, thawed)
- ½ cup of black beans, drained and rinsed
- 1 avocado, diced
- ¼ cup of chopped cilantro
- Lime wedges for serving

For the Dressing:

- 2 **tbsp.** lime juice
- 2 **tbsp.** olive oil
- 1 clove garlic, minced
- Salt and pepper to taste

Instructions:

1. Coat the shrimp well in olive oil, then add chili powder, cumin, garlic powder, salt, and pepper. Toss to coat.
2. Bring a skillet to a medium-high temperature. When the shrimp are pink and opaque throughout, add the seasoning and cook for two to three minutes on each side.
3. Toss together the salad greens, corn, black beans, cilantro, avocado, and halved cherry tomatoes in a big bowl.

4. To prepare the dressing, combine the lime juice, olive oil, minced garlic, salt, and pepper in a small bowl and whisk to combine.
5. Paste the shrimp that have been cooked into the salad.
6. After you've drizzled the dressing over the salad, toss it to cover all the ingredients.
7. Garnish with lime wedges and serve right away.

Nutrition Information (per serving):

Calories: 320

Total Fat: 18g

Cholesterol: 200mg

Sodium: 340mg

Total Carbohydrates: 17g

Dietary Fiber: 7g

Sugars: 3g

Protein: 26g

Kale and Cranberry Salad

Prep Time: 15 minutes

Cook Time: 0 minutes

Servings: 4

Ingredients:

- 1 bunch kale, stems removed and leaves chopped
- ¼ cup of dried cranberries
- ¼ cup of sliced almonds, toasted
- ¼ cup of crumbled feta cheese
- ¼ cup of extra virgin olive oil
- 2 **tbsp.** apple cider vinegar
- 1 **tsp** honey
- Salt and pepper to taste

Instructions:

1. Grind the feta cheese into the chopped greens, add the dried cranberries and toasted sliced almonds to a big mixing basin.
2. The dressing is made by whisking together raw honey, apple cider vinegar, extra virgin olive oil, salt, and pepper in a small bowl.
3. After combining the salad components, pour the dressing over them and mix well.
4. To make the tastes more harmonious, serve right away or let sit in the fridge for at least one or two hours.

Nutrition Information (per serving):

Calories: 220

Total Fat: 16g

Cholesterol: 5mg

Sodium: 180mg

Total Carbohydrates: 17g

Dietary Fiber: 2g

Sugars: 8g

Protein: 4g

Greek Salad with Feta and Olives

Prep Time: 15 minutes

Cook Time: 0 minutes

Servings: 4

Ingredients:

- 4 cups of mixed salad greens
- 1 cucumber, diced
- 1 bell pepper, diced
- 1 cup of cherry tomatoes, halved
- ½ red onion, thinly sliced
- ¼ cup of Kalamata olives, pitted and halved
- ¼ cup of crumbled feta cheese
- 2 **tbsp.** extra virgin olive oil
- 1 tbsp. red wine vinegar
- 1 **tsp** dried oregano
- Salt and pepper to taste

Instructions:

1. Toss together leafy greens, diced cucumber and bell pepper, chopped cherry tomatoes, thinly sliced red onion, chopped Kalamata olives, crumbled feta cheese, and a large mixing basin.
2. The dressing is made by whisking together red wine vinegar, dried oregano, salt, pepper, extra virgin olive oil, and a small bowl.
3. After combining the salad components, pour the dressing over them and mix well.
4. Quickly serve as a revitalizing appetizer or accompaniment.

Nutrition Information (per serving):

Calories: 150

Total Fat: 11g

Cholesterol: 10mg

Sodium: 250mg

Total Carbohydrates: 12g

Dietary Fiber: 3g

Sugars: 6g

Protein: 4g

Zucchini Noodle Caprese Salad

Prep Time: 15 minutes

Cook Time: 0 minutes

Servings: 4

Ingredients:

- 2 medium zucchinis
- 1 cup of cherry tomatoes, halved
- 1 ball fresh mozzarella cheese, diced
- Fresh basil leaves, chopped
- 2 **tbsp.** extra virgin olive oil
- 1 tbsp. balsamic vinegar
- Salt and pepper to taste
- Balsamic glaze (optional, for drizzling)

Instructions:

1. Zoodles, or zucchini noodles, may be made by spiralizing zucchini.
2. Put the zucchini noodles, cherry tomatoes (halved), fresh mozzarella cheese (diced), and basil leaves (chopped) into a big mixing basin.
3. Dressing: In a small bowl, mix together balsamic vinegar and extra virgin olive oil.
4. After combining the salad components, pour the dressing over them and mix well.
5. Add salt and pepper according to your preference.
6. Quickly serve with a drizzle of balsamic glaze for more taste.

Nutrition Information (per serving):

Calories: 150

Total Fat: 11g

Cholesterol: 15mg

Sodium: 180mg

Total Carbohydrates: 7g

Dietary Fiber: 2g

Sugars: 5g

Protein: 8g

Berry Spinach Salad with Poppy Seed Dressing

Prep Time: 10 minutes

Cook Time: 0 minutes

Servings: 4

Ingredients:

- 6 cups of baby spinach leaves
- 1 cup of mixed berries (such as strawberries, blueberries, raspberries)
- ¼ cup of sliced almonds, toasted
- ¼ cup of crumbled feta cheese
- 2 **tbsp.** extra virgin olive oil
- 2 **tbsp.** balsamic vinegar
- 1 tbsp. honey
- 1 **tsp** Dijon mustard
- 1 **tsp** poppy seeds
- Salt and pepper to taste

Instructions:

1. Toss together the crumbled feta cheese, mixed berries, toasted sliced almonds, and baby spinach leaves in a large mixing basin.
2. To prepare the dressing, combine the poppy seeds, balsamic vinegar, honey, Dijon mustard, extra virgin olive oil, salt, and pepper in a small bowl. Whisk until well combined.
3. After combining the salad components, pour the dressing over them and mix well.
4. For a healthy and revitalizing salad, serve right away.

Nutrition Information (per serving):

Calories: 180

Total Fat: 12g

Cholesterol: 5mg

Sodium: 170mg

Total Carbohydrates: 15g

Dietary Fiber: 4g

Sugars: 9g

Turkey and Avocado Cobb Salad

Prep Time: 15 minutes

Cook Time: 15 minutes

Servings: 4

Ingredients:

- 8 cups of mixed salad greens
- 1 lb. turkey breast, cooked and diced
- 4 slices bacon, cooked and crumbled
- 2 hard-boiled eggs, chopped
- 1 avocado, diced

- 1 cup of cherry tomatoes, halved
- ½ cup of crumbled blue cheese
- ¼ cup of sliced green onions
- Salt and pepper to taste
- Ranch dressing or your favorite dressing, for serving

Instructions:

1. Arrange a bed of mixed salad greens in a big serving basin.
2. Put the salad greens in a row and top it with chopped hard-boiled eggs, crumbled bacon, chopped avocado, halved cherry tomatoes, crumbled blue cheese, and sliced green onions.
3. Add salt and pepper according to your preference.
4. Accompany with ranch dressing or your preferred dressing and serve right away.

Nutrition Information (per serving):

Calories: 380

Total Fat: 23g

Cholesterol: 150mg

Sodium: 650mg

Total Carbohydrates: 9g

Dietary Fiber: 4g

Sugars: 3g

Protein: 35g

Watermelon and Feta Salad

Prep Time: 15 minutes

Cook Time: 0 minutes

Servings: 4

Ingredients:

- 4 cups of cubed watermelon
- ½ cup of crumbled feta cheese
- ¼ cup of sliced red onion
- ¼ cup of chopped fresh mint leaves
- ¼ cup of sliced almonds, toasted
- 2 **tbsp.** extra virgin olive oil
- 1 tbsp. balsamic vinegar
- Salt and pepper to taste

Instructions:

1. Cubes of watermelon, crumbled feta cheese, red onion, chopped mint leaves, and roasted almonds should be combined in a big mixing basin.

2. The dressing is made by whisking together salt, pepper, balsamic vinegar, extra virgin olive oil, and a small bowl.
3. After you've drizzled the dressing over the salad components, gently toss them to cover them evenly.
4. Quickly serve as a colorful and revitalizing salad alternative.

Nutrition Information (per serving):

Calories: 180

Total Fat: 12g

Cholesterol: 10mg

Sodium: 220mg

Total Carbohydrates: 16g

Dietary Fiber: 2g

Sugars: 12g

Protein: 4g

Apple Pecan Chicken Salad

Prep Time: 15 minutes

Cook Time: 15 minutes (if cooking chicken)

Servings: 4

Ingredients:

- 2 boneless, skinless chicken breasts, cooked and diced
- 2 apples, diced
- ½ cup of chopped pecans, toasted
- ¼ cup of diced celery
- ¼ cup of dried cranberries
- ¼ cup of mayonnaise
- 2 **tbsp.** Greek yogurt
- 1 tbsp. lemon juice
- 1 **tsp** honey
- Salt and pepper to taste
- Mixed salad greens for serving

Instructions:

1. Get a big bowl and throw in some cooked chicken breasts, apples, roasted walnuts, celery, and dried cranberries. Chop them up and mix them together.
2. The dressing is made by whisking together mayonnaise, Greek yogurt, honey, lemon juice, salt, and pepper in a small bowl.
3. Toss the salad components with the dressing until they are well covered.
4. Spoon onto a mixture of salad greens.

Nutrition Information (per serving, excluding salad greens):

Calories: 350

Total Fat: 22g

Cholesterol: 70mg

Sodium: 200mg

Total Carbohydrates: 24g

Dietary Fiber: 4g

Sugars: 18g

Protein: 18g

Broccoli and Bacon Salad

Prep Time: 15 minutes

Cook Time: 0 minutes

Servings: 4

Ingredients:

- 4 cups of broccoli florets
- 4 slices bacon, cooked and crumbled
- ¼ cup of diced red onion
- ¼ cup of raisins or dried cranberries
- ¼ cup of chopped walnuts, toasted
- ½ cup of mayonnaise
- 2 **tbsp.** apple cider vinegar
- 1 tbsp. honey
- Salt and pepper to taste

Instructions:

1. Toss the broccoli florets with the crumbled cooked bacon, sliced red onion, chopped toasted walnuts, raisins, or dried cranberries in a large mixing dish.
2. The dressing is made by whisking together mayonnaise, honey, apple cider vinegar, salt, and pepper in a small bowl.
3. Toss the salad components with the dressing until they are well covered.
4. Refrigerate until serving time or serve immediately.

Nutrition Information (per serving):

Calories: 320

Total Fat: 26g

Cholesterol: 20mg

Sodium: 350mg

Total Carbohydrates: 18g

Dietary Fiber: 4g

Sugars: 10g

Protein: 7g

Tuna and White Bean Salad

Prep Time: 10 minutes

Cook Time: 0 minutes

Servings: 4

Ingredients:

- 2 cans (5 oz. each) tuna, drained
- 1 can (15 oz.) white beans (cannellini or Great Northern), drained and rinsed
- ¼ cup of diced red onion
- ¼ cup of chopped fresh parsley
- 2 **tbsp.** extra virgin olive oil
- 1 tbsp. lemon juice
- 1 **tsp** Dijon mustard
- Salt and pepper to taste
- Mixed salad greens for serving

Instructions:

1. Mix together the white beans, drained and rinsed, diced red onion, chopped fresh parsley, and drained tuna in a large mixing dish.
2. The dressing is made by whisking together salt, pepper, lemon juice, Dijon mustard, and extra virgin olive oil in a small bowl.
3. Toss the salad components with the dressing until they are well covered.
4. Spoon onto a mixture of salad greens.

Nutrition Information (per serving, excluding salad greens):

Calories: 250

Total Fat: 8g

Cholesterol: 25mg

Sodium: 400mg

Total Carbohydrates: 20g

Dietary Fiber: 6g

Sugars: 1g

Protein: 22g

FISH & SEAFOOD

Lemon Garlic Shrimp Scampi

Prep Time: 10 minutes

Cook Time: 10 minutes

Servings: 4

Ingredients:

- 1 lb. large shrimp, peeled and deveined
- 4 **tbsp.** unsalted butter
- 4 cloves garlic, minced
- Zest of 1 lemon
- Juice of 1 lemon
- ¼ cup of white wine (optional)
- Salt and pepper to taste
- 2 **tbsp.** chopped fresh parsley
- Cooked pasta or crusty bread for serving (optional)

Instructions:

1. Butter should be melted in a big pan over medium heat. If using minced garlic, sauté for about 1 minute or until aromatic.
2. Sauté the shrimp for two or three minutes on each side, or until they become pink.
3. Add the zest, juice, and (if using) white wine of the lemons. Just a minute or two will do it.
4. Add salt and pepper according to your preference. Combine with the freshly cut parsley.
5. If you like, you may top it with cooked spaghetti or serve it hot with some crusty toast.

Nutrition Information (per serving):

Calories: 220

Total Fat: 13g

Cholesterol: 200mg

Sodium: 280mg

Total Carbohydrates: 3g

Dietary Fiber: 0g

Sugars: 0g

Protein: 21g

Grilled Salmon with Dill Sauce

Prep Time: 10 minutes

Cook Time: 10 minutes

Servings: 4

Ingredients:

- 4 salmon fillets (about 6 oz. each)
- Salt and pepper to taste

- 2 **tbsp.** olive oil
- ¼ cup of plain Greek yogurt
- 2 **tbsp.** chopped fresh dill
- 1 tbsp. lemon juice
- 1 clove garlic, minced
- 1 **tsp** Dijon mustard

Instructions:

1. Warm up the grill to a medium-high temperature.
2. Before drizzling olive oil over the salmon fillets, season them with salt and pepper.
3. Grill the salmon fillets for four to five minutes on each side, or until they achieve the doneness you choose.
4. The dill sauce is made by combining Greek yogurt, chopped fresh dill, lemon juice, minced garlic, and Dijon mustard in a small bowl.
5. Top grilled salmon with dill sauce and serve hot.

Nutrition Information (per serving):

Calories: 350

Total Fat: 21g

Cholesterol: 100mg

Sodium: 120mg

Total Carbohydrates: 1g

Dietary Fiber: 0g

Sugars: 0g

Protein: 36g

Cajun Blackened Tilapia

Prep Time: 10 minutes

Cook Time: 10 minutes

Servings: 4

Ingredients:

- 4 tilapia fillets
- 2 **tbsp.** Cajun seasoning
- 2 **tbsp.** olive oil
- 1 tbsp. butter
- Lemon wedges for serving

Instructions:

1. Use paper towels to gently pat dry the fillets of tilapia.
2. Coat each fillet equally with Cajun seasoning.
3. In a large pan, melt the butter and olive oil over medium-high heat.
4. Cook the tilapia fillets for three to four minutes each side, or until they are opaque throughout and have a little charred, once the pan has heated.
5. Warm the dish and garnish with lemon wedges.

Nutrition Information (per serving):

Calories: 220

Total Fat: 12g

Cholesterol: 60mg

Sodium: 350mg

Total Carbohydrates: 2g

Dietary Fiber: 1g

Sugars: 0g

Protein: 25g

<u>Teriyaki Glazed Mahi Mahi</u>

Prep Time: 10 minutes

Cook Time: 15 minutes

Servings: 4

Ingredients:

- 4 Mahi Mahi fillets
- ¼ cup of soy sauce
- 2 **tbsp.** honey
- 2 **tbsp.** rice vinegar
- 1 clove garlic, minced
- 1 **tsp** grated ginger
- 1 tbsp. sesame oil
- 2 **tbsp.** chopped green onions (for garnish)
- Sesame seeds (for garnish)

Instructions:

1. To prepare the teriyaki glaze, combine the following ingredients in a bowl: rice vinegar, soy sauce, honey, grated ginger, garlic, and sesame oil. Whisk until well combined.
2. Place a grill or pan on a medium-high heat burner.
3. Grill the Mahi Mahi fillets for 5 to 6 minutes each side, or until the fish flakes easily when tested with a fork.
4. As the Mahi Mahi fillets are nearing the end of their grilling time, brush them with the teriyaki sauce and let it caramelize a little.
5. After taking it off the grill, spice it up with some sesame seeds and chopped green onions.
6. Keep warm before serving.

Nutrition Information (per serving):

Calories: 250

Total Fat: 5g

Cholesterol: 125mg

Sodium: 600mg

Total Carbohydrates: 10g

Dietary Fiber: 0g

Sugars: 9g

Protein: 40g

Baked Cod with Herb Crust

Prep Time: 10 minutes

Cook Time: 15 minutes

Servings: 4

Ingredients:

- 4 cod fillets
- Salt and pepper to taste
- 2 **tbsp.** olive oil
- ½ cup of breadcrumbs
- 2 **tbsp.** chopped fresh parsley
- 1 tbsp. chopped fresh dill
- 1 tbsp. chopped fresh chives
- 2 cloves garlic, minced
- Zest of 1 lemon
- Lemon wedges for serving

Instructions:

1. Set the oven temperature to 400°F, or 200°C. Gather parchment paper and set it aside.
2. After seasoning the cod fillets with salt and pepper, pat them dry with paper towels.
3. The fresh parsley, dill, chives, breadcrumbs, garlic, and zest of the lemon should all be combined in a bowl.
4. Apply a little olive oil to the surface of each cod fillet, and then press the herb breadcrumb mixture firmly onto it.
5. Once the baking sheet is ready, add the cod fillets and bake for 12–15 minutes, or until the fish flakes readily when tested with a fork.
6. Warm the dish and garnish with lemon wedges.

Nutrition Information (per serving):

Calories: 250

Total Fat: 9g

Cholesterol: 60mg

Sodium: 300mg

Total Carbohydrates: 10g

Dietary Fiber: 1g

Sugars: 1g

Protein: 30g

Garlic Butter Shrimp Skewers

Prep Time: 10 minutes

Cook Time: 5 minutes

Servings: 4

Ingredients:

- 1 lb. large shrimp, peeled and deveined
- 4 cloves garlic, minced
- ¼ cup of unsalted butter, melted
- 2 **tbsp.** chopped fresh parsley
- 1 tbsp. lemon juice
- Salt and pepper to taste
- Lemon wedges for serving

Instructions:

1. Warm up the grill to a medium-high temperature. Soaking wooden skewers in water for 30 minutes can keep them from burning.
2. Toss together the butter, parsley, garlic, lemon juice, salt, and pepper in a bowl.
3. The shrimp should be threaded onto skewers.
4. Dip the shrimp skewers in the garlic butter mixture on both sides.
5. To get a pink and opaque shrimp color, grill the skewers for two to three minutes each side.
6. Warm the dish and garnish with lemon wedges.

Nutrition Information (per serving):

Calories: 180

Total Fat: 12g

Cholesterol: 160mg

Sodium: 200mg

Total Carbohydrates: 2g

Dietary Fiber: 0g

Sugars: 0g

Protein: 16g

Thai Coconut Curry Shrimp

Prep Time: 10 minutes

Cook Time: 15 minutes

Servings: 4

Ingredients:

- 1 lb. large shrimp, peeled and deveined
- 1 tbsp. coconut oil
- 1 onion, finely chopped
- 2 cloves garlic, minced
- 1 red bell pepper, sliced
- 1 yellow bell pepper, sliced
- 1 can (14 oz.) coconut milk
- 2 **tbsp.** Thai red curry paste

- 1 tbsp. fish sauce
- 1 tbsp. brown sugar
- 1 tbsp. lime juice
- Salt and pepper to taste
- Fresh cilantro leaves for garnish
- Cooked rice or noodles for serving

Instructions:

1. Turn the heat up to medium in a big skillet and add the coconut oil. Sauté the minced garlic and diced onion until they release their aroma.
2. Toss in some sliced red and yellow bell peppers and sauté for a couple of minutes, or until they begin to soften a little.
3. Coat the mixture with brown sugar, fish sauce, red curry pastes from Thailand, and coconut milk. Simmer the ingredients for a while.
4. Sauté the shrimp in a pan after peeling and deveining them for 5 to 6 minutes, or until they become pink and are opaque throughout.
5. Add the lime juice and add salt and pepper according to your taste.
6. Hot, topped with cooked rice or noodles and a sprinkle of fresh cilantro leaves, serve.

Nutrition Information (per serving, without rice or noodles):

Calories: 280

Total Fat: 20g

Cholesterol: 170mg

Sodium: 420mg

Total Carbohydrates: 10g

Dietary Fiber: 2g

Sugars: 5g

Protein: 18g

Lemon Herb Baked Trout

Prep Time: 10 minutes

Cook Time: 15 minutes

Servings: 4

Ingredients:

- 4 trout fillets
- Salt and pepper to taste
- 2 **tbsp.** olive oil
- 2 cloves garlic, minced
- Zest of 1 lemon
- 1 tbsp. chopped fresh parsley
- 1 tbsp. chopped fresh dill
- Lemon slices for garnish

Instructions:

1. Set the oven temperature to 400°F, or 200°C. Gather parchment paper and set it aside.
2. Use paper towels to pat the fish fillets dry, then season with salt and pepper.
3. To make the dressing, combine the olive oil, garlic powder, lemon zest, parsley, and dill in a small bowl.
4. Arrange the fillets of fish on the baking sheet that has been preheated. Coat the fillets with the herb mixture using a brush.
5. Cook the fish for 12–15 minutes in a preheated oven, or until it flakes easily when tested with a fork.
6. Warm and serve with lemon wedges as a garnish.

Nutrition Information (per serving):

Calories: 220

Total Fat: 13g

Cholesterol: 60mg

Sodium: 75mg

Total Carbohydrates: 1g

Dietary Fiber: 0g

Sugars: 0g

Protein: 23g

<u>Spicy Sriracha Lime Grilled Shrimp</u>

Prep Time: 15 minutes

Cook Time: 5 minutes

Servings: 4

Ingredients:

- 1 lb. large shrimp, peeled and deveined
- 2 **tbsp.** Sriracha sauce
- 2 **tbsp.** olive oil
- Zest and juice of 1 lime
- 2 cloves garlic, minced
- 1 tbsp. honey
- Salt and pepper to taste
- Lime wedges and chopped cilantro for garnish

Instructions:

1. Combine the Sriracha sauce, olive oil, fresh lime juice and zest, garlic powder, honey, salt, and pepper in a mixing bowl.
2. Coat the shrimp equally by adding them to the bowl after peeling and deveining them.
3. Warm up the grill to a medium-high temperature.

4. If you're using skewers, thread the shrimp onto them.
5. To get a pinkish hue and fully cooked shrimp, grill for two to three minutes each side.
6. After taking it off the grill, place lime wedges and chopped cilantro on top.
7. Keep warm before serving.

Nutrition Information (per serving):

Calories: 180

Total Fat: 9g

Cholesterol: 170mg

Sodium: 280mg

Total Carbohydrates: 5g

Dietary Fiber: 0g

Sugars: 3g

Protein: 20g

Mediterranean Baked Halibut

Prep Time: 10 minutes

Cook Time: 15 minutes

Servings: 4

Ingredients:

- 4 halibut fillets
- Salt and pepper to taste
- 2 **tbsp.** olive oil
- 4 cloves garlic, minced
- 1 cup of cherry tomatoes, halved
- ¼ cup of Kalamata olives, pitted and halved
- 2 **tbsp.** capers
- 1 tbsp. chopped fresh parsley
- 1 tbsp. chopped fresh basil
- 1 tbsp. lemon juice

Instructions:

1. Set the oven temperature to 400°F, or 200°C. Parchment paper should be lined into a baking dish.
2. After removing excess moisture with paper towels, season the halibut fillets with salt and pepper.
3. Melt the olive oil in a pan set over medium heat. Sauté the minced garlic until it releases its aroma.
4. Toss in capers, cherry tomatoes, and Kalamata olives, all halved. Be sure to cook for two or three minutes.
5. After you have the baking dish ready, lay the halibut fillets on top. Spoon the

fillets with the olive, tomato, and garlic mixture.

6. Cook the fish for 12–15 minutes in a preheated oven, or until it flakes easily when tested with a fork.
7. Take it out and top it with some fresh basil and parsley that you cut up. Serve with a drizzle of lemon juice.

Nutrition Information (per serving):

Calories: 250

Total Fat: 12g

Cholesterol: 60mg

Sodium: 450mg

Total Carbohydrates: 6g

Dietary Fiber: 2g

Sugars: 2g

Protein: 30g

CHICKEN

Balsamic Glazed Chicken Breast

Prep Time: 10 minutes

Cook Time: 20 minutes

Servings: 4

Ingredients:

- 4 boneless, skinless chicken breasts
- Salt and pepper to taste
- 2 **tbsp.** olive oil
- ¼ cup of balsamic vinegar
- 2 **tbsp.** honey
- 2 cloves garlic, minced
- 1 **tsp** dried basil
- 1 **tsp** dried oregano
- ½ **tsp** dried thyme
- Fresh parsley for garnish (optional)

Instructions:

1. Turn the oven on high heat (375°F, 190°C).
2. Put some salt and pepper on the chicken breasts and season them both sides.
3. Brown the olive oil in a pan that may be placed in the oven on medium-high heat.
4. Brown the chicken breasts by adding them to the pan and cooking for two or three minutes each side.

5. In a little basin, combine the balsamic vinegar, honey, minced garlic, dried basil, dried oregano, and dried thyme. Whisk to combine.
6. Once the chicken breasts are browned in the pan, pour the balsamic mixture over them.
7. When the chicken reaches an internal temperature of 165°F (75°C), remove it from the pan and place it in the preheated oven. Bake for 15-20 minutes, or until done.
8. Before serving, garnish with fresh parsley if preferred.

Nutrition Information (per serving):

Calories: 250

Total Fat: 9g

Cholesterol: 80mg

Sodium: 150mg

Total Carbohydrates: 8g

Dietary Fiber: 0g

Sugars: 7g

Protein: 31g

Skinny Chicken Alfredo

Prep Time: 10 minutes

Cook Time: 20 minutes

Servings: 4

Ingredients:

- 8 oz. whole wheat fettuccine
- 2 boneless, skinless chicken breasts, cut into strips
- Salt and pepper to taste
- 1 tbsp. olive oil
- 2 cloves garlic, minced
- 1 cup of low-fat milk
- 1 tbsp. cornstarch
- ¼ cup of grated Parmesan cheese
- 1 tbsp. chopped fresh parsley
- Optional: steamed vegetables for serving

Instructions:

1. Fettuccine should be cooked following the directions on the box. Reserve the drained liquid.
2. Add salt and pepper to the chicken strips.
3. In a big skillet, heat the olive oil over medium heat. Sauté the minced garlic until it releases its aroma.
4. Brown the chicken strips in a pan over medium heat, stirring occasionally, for 5 to 6 minutes on each side, or until done.

5. Whisk the cornstarch and low-fat milk together well in a small bowl.
6. Add the cooked chicken to the pan with the milk mixture. In approximately three or four minutes, while stirring constantly, the sauce should thicken.
7. Melt the grated Parmesan cheese in the pan and toss it into the sauce.
8. Before tossing in the cooked fettuccine, be sure to cover it well with the sauce in the pan.
9. Serve with a sprinkle of chopped fresh parsley. Whether you like it hot or cold, serve with steamed veggies.

Nutrition Information (per serving):

Calories: 350

Total Fat: 9g

Cholesterol: 60mg

Sodium: 250mg

Total Carbohydrates: 35g

Dietary Fiber: 5g

Sugars: 4g

Protein: 32g

Lemon Herb Roasted Chicken Thighs

Prep Time: 10 minutes

Cook Time: 35 minutes

Servings: 4

Ingredients:

- 8 bone-in, skin-on chicken thighs
- Salt and pepper to taste
- 2 **tbsp.** olive oil
- Zest and juice of 1 lemon
- 2 cloves garlic, minced
- 1 **tsp** dried thyme
- 1 **tsp** dried rosemary
- 1 **tsp** dried oregano
- Fresh parsley for garnish (optional)

Instructions:

1. Set the oven temperature to 400°F, or 200°C. Gather parchment paper and set it aside.
2. Use paper towels to pat the chicken thighs dry, then season with pepper and salt.
3. Blend the olive oil, lemon zest and juice, minced garlic, dried thyme, rosemary, and oregano in a small bowl.

4. Coat the chicken thighs equally with the herb and lemon mixture.
5. Arrange the chicken thighs on the baking sheet that has been preheated.
6. Once the oven is hot, roast the chicken for 30–35 minutes, or until it reaches a temperature of 165°F (75°C) throughout.
7. Before serving, garnish with fresh parsley.

Nutrition Information (per serving):

Calories: 380

Total Fat: 25g

Cholesterol: 160mg

Sodium: 280mg

Total Carbohydrates: 1g

Dietary Fiber: 0g

Sugars: 0g

Protein: 36g

BBQ Chicken Lettuce Wraps

Prep Time: 15 minutes

Cook Time: 15 minutes

Servings: 4

Ingredients:

- 1 lb. boneless, skinless chicken breasts, cut into small pieces
- Salt and pepper to taste
- 1 tbsp. olive oil
- ½ cup of barbecue sauce
- ¼ cup of diced red onion
- ¼ cup of diced bell pepper
- ¼ cup of diced tomatoes
- ¼ cup of corn kernels (fresh, frozen, or canned)
- ¼ cup of black beans (canned), drained and rinsed
- ¼ cup of chopped fresh cilantro
- Iceberg or butter lettuce leaves for wrapping

Instructions:

1. Add salt and pepper to the chicken pieces.
2. In a pan set over medium-high heat, warm the olive oil. Once the chicken is browned and cooked through, add the pieces and simmer for another five to seven minutes.
3. Turn the stove down to low and coat the pan with barbecue sauce. To make sure the chicken is covered evenly, stir in the sauce. Just

a few more minutes of cooking time.

4. Turn off the stove and mix in the diced tomatoes, bell pepper, corn, black beans, and chopped cilantro with the diced red onion and bell pepper.
5. Before serving, roll up some lettuce leaves and ladle on some BBQ chicken mixture.
6. Make sure to serve right away.

Nutrition Information (per serving):

Calories: 280

Total Fat: 7g

Cholesterol: 75mg

Sodium: 450mg

Total Carbohydrates: 22g

Dietary Fiber: 3g

Sugars: 14g

Protein: 31g

<u>Honey Mustard Chicken Skewers</u>

Prep Time: 15 minutes

Cook Time: 10 minutes

Servings: 4

Ingredients:

- 1 lb. boneless, skinless chicken breasts, cut into cubes
- Salt and pepper to taste
- ¼ cup of honey
- 2 **tbsp.** Dijon mustard
- 1 tbsp. olive oil
- 2 cloves garlic, minced
- Wooden skewers, soaked in water for 30 minutes

Instructions:

1. After cubing the chicken, season it with salt & pepper.
2. Beets, Dijon mustard, olive oil, and garlic powder should be mixed in a basin.
3. Thread the moistened wooden skewers with the chicken chunks.
4. Distribute the honey mustard mixture evenly over the chicken skewers by brushing it on.
5. Set the grill or pan over medium-high heat to get it hot.
6. To make sure the chicken is cooked through and no longer pink in the middle, grill the skewers for four to five minutes each side.
7. Keep warm before serving.

Nutrition Information (per serving):

Calories: 250

Total Fat: 7g

Cholesterol: 75mg

Sodium: 250mg

Total Carbohydrates: 17g

Dietary Fiber: 0g

Sugars: 16g

Protein: 28g

Greek Yogurt Parmesan Crusted Chicken

Prep Time: 15 minutes

Cook Time: 20 minutes

Servings: 4

Ingredients:

- 4 boneless, skinless chicken breasts
- Salt and pepper to taste
- ½ cup of plain Greek yogurt
- ¼ cup of grated Parmesan cheese
- ½ **tsp** garlic powder
- ½ **tsp** onion powder
- ½ **tsp** paprika
- ¼ **tsp** dried thyme
- Cooking spray

Instructions:

1. Set the oven temperature to 400°F, or 200°C. Gather parchment paper and set it aside.
2. Season the chicken breasts with pepper and salt.
3. Garlic powder, onion powder, paprika, dried thyme, shredded Parmesan cheese, Greek yogurt, and combine in a small basin.
4. Coat both sides of each chicken breast with the yogurt mixture.
5. Once the baking sheet is ready, set the breaded chicken breasts on top.
6. The chicken should be cooked through and the crust should be golden brown after 18 to 20 minutes in a preheated oven.
7. Keep warm before serving.

Nutrition Information (per serving):

Calories: 280

Total Fat: 9g

Cholesterol: 90mg

Sodium: 250mg

Total Carbohydrates: 3g

Dietary Fiber: 0g

Sugars: 2g

Protein: 43g

Mango Salsa Chicken

Prep Time: 15 minutes

Cook Time: 20 minutes

Servings: 4

Ingredients:

- 4 boneless, skinless chicken breasts
- Salt and pepper to taste
- 1 tbsp. olive oil
- 1 mango, peeled and diced
- ½ red bell pepper, diced
- ¼ cup of diced red onion
- 1 jalapeño, seeded and diced
- Juice of 1 lime
- 2 **tbsp.** chopped fresh cilantro
- Cooking spray

Instructions:

1. Set the grill or pan over medium-high heat to get it hot.
2. Season the chicken breasts with pepper and salt.
3. Coat the chicken breasts with olive oil.
4. Chicken breasts should be grilled for about seven or eight minutes each side, or until done and no longer pink in the middle.
5. To create the salsa, put the diced mango, red bell pepper, red onion, jalapeño, lime juice, and chopped cilantro into a bowl.
6. Mango salsa is a delicious topping for grilled chicken breasts.

Nutrition Information (per serving):

Calories: 280

Total Fat: 9g

Cholesterol: 90mg

Sodium: 250mg

Total Carbohydrates: 12g

Dietary Fiber: 2g

Sugars: 8g

Protein: 38g

Buffalo Chicken Stuffed Sweet Potatoes

Prep Time: 10 minutes

Cook Time: 1 hour

Servings: 4

Ingredients:

- 4 medium sweet potatoes

- 2 cups of shredded cooked chicken
- ½ cup of buffalo sauce
- ¼ cup of ranch dressing
- ¼ cup of chopped green onions
- ¼ cup of crumbled blue cheese (optional)
- Salt and pepper to taste

Instructions:

1. Set the oven temperature to 400°F, or 200°C.
2. After washing, make many holes in sweet potatoes with a fork. Arrange them on a parchment-lined baking sheet.
3. Once the oven is hot, bake the sweet potatoes for 45 to 60 minutes, or until they are soft.
4. Whisk together the cooked chicken, ranch dressing, buffalo sauce, and shredded chicken in a bowl.
5. After cooking sweet potatoes, let them to cool for a little before slicing them lengthwise.
6. Divide the buffalo chicken mixture among the sweet potatoes and stuff them.
7. For an optional garnish of crumbled blue cheese and chopped green onions, serve.
8. Add salt and pepper according to your preference.
9. Keep warm before serving.

Nutrition Information (per serving):

Calories: 350

Total Fat: 10g

Cholesterol: 80mg

Sodium: 950mg

Total Carbohydrates: 42g

Dietary Fiber: 6g

Sugars: 9g

Protein: 25g

Pesto Chicken with Roasted Vegetables

Prep Time: 15 minutes

Cook Time: 25 minutes

Servings: 4

Ingredients:

- 4 boneless, skinless chicken breasts
- Salt and pepper to taste
- ¼ cup of prepared pesto sauce

- 2 cups of mixed vegetables (such as cherry tomatoes, bell peppers, zucchini, and red onion), chopped
- 2 **tbsp.** olive oil
- 2 cloves garlic, minced
- 1 tbsp. balsamic vinegar
- Fresh basil leaves for garnish

Instructions:

1. Set the oven temperature to 400°F, or 200°C.
2. Season the chicken breasts with pepper and salt.
3. After seasoning the chicken breasts, coat them equally with pesto sauce.
4. Toss the mixed veggies in a basin with the olive oil, balsamic vinegar, and minced garlic until well covered.
5. On a parchment-lined baking sheet, spread the chicken breasts and veggies.
6. The chicken should be cooked thoroughly and the veggies should be soft after 20 to 25 minutes in a preheated oven.
7. Prior to serving, top with a few fresh basil leaves.
8. Keep warm before serving.

Nutrition Information (per serving):

Calories: 320

Total Fat: 15g

Cholesterol: 80mg

Sodium: 380mg

Total Carbohydrates: 9g

Dietary Fiber: 3g

Sugars: 4g

Protein: 35g

Chicken and Broccoli Stir-Fry

Prep Time: 15 minutes

Cook Time: 15 minutes

Servings: 4

Ingredients:

- 1 lb. boneless, skinless chicken breasts, sliced
- Salt and pepper to taste
- 2 **tbsp.** soy sauce
- 1 tbsp. hoisin sauce
- 1 tbsp. oyster sauce
- 2 **tbsp.** vegetable oil
- 2 cloves garlic, minced
- 1 **tsp** grated ginger
- 2 cups of broccoli florets
- 1 bell pepper, sliced

- 1 onion, sliced
- Cooked rice for serving

Instructions:

1. Pepper and salt the chicken slices.
2. Combine the oyster sauce, hoisin sauce, and soy sauce in a small bowl.
3. In a big wok or pan set over medium-high heat, warm the vegetable oil.
4. After 30 seconds of stirring, add the grated ginger and minced garlic to the pan.
5. In a pan over medium heat, brown the chicken pieces and cook them until done.
6. Set aside the chicken after removing it from the pan.
7. Chop some onion and bell pepper and toss them in with the broccoli florets in the same pan. Cook the veggies in a skillet until they are crisp-tender.
8. Put the cooked chicken back into the pan.
9. After mixing the sauce ingredients, pour them over the chicken and veggies. For a uniform coating, give everything a good stir.
10. Stir periodically and continue cooking for another two to three minutes.
11. Top with cooked rice and serve hot.

Nutrition Information (per serving, excluding rice):

Calories: 280

Total Fat: 14g

Cholesterol: 80mg

Sodium: 550mg

Total Carbohydrates: 9g

Dietary Fiber: 3g

Sugars: 4g

Protein: 30g

BEEF, PORK

Beef and Broccoli Stir-Fry

Prep Time: 15 minutes

Cook Time: 15 minutes

Servings: 4

Ingredients:

- 1 lb. beef sirloin or flank steak, thinly sliced
- Salt and pepper to taste
- ¼ cup of soy sauce
- 2 **tbsp.** oyster sauce
- 1 tbsp. hoisin sauce
- 1 tbsp. sesame oil
- 2 **tbsp.** vegetable oil
- 3 cloves garlic, minced
- 1 **tsp** grated ginger
- 4 cups of broccoli florets
- Cooked rice for serving
- Sesame seeds for garnish (optional)

Instructions:

1. Rub thinly sliced meat with pepper and salt.
2. Combine the sesame oil, hoisin sauce, oyster sauce, and soy sauce in a small bowl.
3. In a big wok or pan set over medium-high heat, warm the vegetable oil.
4. After 30 seconds of stirring, add the grated ginger and minced garlic to the pan.
5. Brown the cut meat by adding it to the skillet.
6. Take the meat out of the pan and put it aside.
7. Cook the broccoli florets until they are almost crisp-tender in the same pan.
8. Bring the steak back to a simmer in the pan.
9. Top the broccoli and meat with the sauce mixture. For a uniform coating, give everything a good stir.
10. Stir periodically and continue cooking for another two to three minutes.
11. Top with cooked rice and serve hot.
12. Sesame seeds may be used as a garnish if preferred.

Nutrition Information (per serving, excluding rice):

Calories: 320

Total Fat: 20g

Cholesterol: 50mg

Sodium: 850mg

Total Carbohydrates: 10g

Dietary Fiber: 3g

Sugars: 3g

Protein: 25g

Korean Beef Bowl

Prep Time: 15 minutes

Cook Time: 15 minutes

Servings: 4

Ingredients:

- 1 lb. ground beef
- ¼ cup of soy sauce
- 2 **tbsp.** brown sugar
- 1 tbsp. sesame oil
- 2 cloves garlic, minced
- 1 **tsp** grated ginger
- 2 green onions, thinly sliced
- Cooked rice for serving
- Sesame seeds for garnish
- Sliced green onions for garnish (optional)

Instructions:

1. Toss the green onions, garlic, brown sugar, sesame oil, and soy sauce in a small bowl. Add the grated ginger and minced garlic.
2. On a medium-high heat, warm a big skillet. Toss in the ground meat and simmer, stirring occasionally, until browned and well cooked.
3. The extra fat should be drained out of the pan.
4. After the ground beef has cooked in the pan, pour the sauce mixture over it. Mix thoroughly.
5. Add a couple of more minutes of cooking time to let the flavors combine.
6. Top with cooked rice and serve hot.
7. If you'd like, you may top it up with chopped green onions and sesame seeds.

Nutrition Information (per serving, excluding rice):

Calories: 350

Total Fat: 20g

Cholesterol: 80mg

Sodium: 800mg

Total Carbohydrates: 10g

Dietary Fiber: 1g

Sugars: 7g

Protein: 30g

Pork Tenderloin with Balsamic Glaze

Prep Time: 10 minutes

Cook Time: 25 minutes

Servings: 4

Ingredients:

- 1 lb. pork tenderloin
- Salt and pepper to taste
- 1 tbsp. olive oil
- ¼ cup of balsamic vinegar
- 2 **tbsp.** honey

- 2 cloves garlic, minced
- ½ cup of chicken broth or stock
- Fresh rosemary or thyme for garnish (optional)

Instructions:

1. Turn the oven on high heat (400°F, 200°C).
2. Rub some salt and pepper onto the pork tenderloin.
3. With an oven-safe skillet set over medium-high heat, warm the olive oil.
4. Grill the pork tenderloin for two or three minutes on each side, or until it becomes a golden brown.
5. Combine the chicken broth, honey, minced garlic, and balsamic vinegar in a small bowl.
6. Once the pork tenderloin is brown in the pan, pour the balsamic mixture over it.
7. Place the pan in the oven and roast for 15 to 20 minutes, or until the pork achieves an internal temperature of 145 degrees Fahrenheit (63 degrees Celsius).
8. Lay the pork tenderloin to rest for a few minutes after removing it from the pan. Then, slice it thinly.
9. In the meanwhile, heat up the skillet over medium heat, adding the pan juices. Keep the sauce simmering until it slightly thickens.
10. Brush the pork tenderloin with balsamic glaze and slice it.
11. If desired, garnish with fresh thyme or rosemary.
12. Keep warm before serving.

Nutrition Information (per serving):

Calories: 250

Total Fat: 8g

Cholesterol: 75mg

Sodium: 300mg

Total Carbohydrates: 10g

Dietary Fiber: 0g

Sugars: 9g

Protein: 30g

Beef Stroganoff

Prep Time: 10 minutes

Cook Time: 20 minutes

Servings: 4

Ingredients:

- 1 lb. beef sirloin, thinly sliced
- Salt and pepper to taste
- 2 **tbsp.** olive oil
- 1 onion, thinly sliced
- 2 cloves garlic, minced
- 8 oz mushrooms, sliced
- 2 **tbsp.** all-purpose flour
- 1 cup of beef broth
- 1 tbsp. Worcestershire sauce
- ½ cup of sour cream
- Cooked egg noodles or rice for serving
- Chopped fresh parsley for garnish (optional)

Instructions:

1. Use salt and pepper to season the thinly cut sirloin of beef.
2. A big skillet with olive oil in it should be heated over medium-high heat.
3. Saute the beef slices for two or three minutes on each side, or until they begin to brown. Take it off the heat and put it aside.
4. Toss in the minced garlic and sliced onions in the same pan. It should take around two or three minutes for the vegetables to soften in the pan.
5. Toss in some sliced mushrooms and sauté them until they shrink a little and give off some moisture.
6. Toss the veggies with the all-purpose flour and give them a good toss.
7. While continually whisking to avoid lumps, slowly add Worcestershire sauce and beef broth.
8. Simmer the ingredients for about 5 minutes, or until the sauce thickens.
9. Stir in the cooked steak before returning it to the pan.
10. Take the pan off the stove and mix in the sour cream until combined.
11. Rice or cooked egg noodles are good accompaniments to beef stroganoff.
12. Chopped fresh parsley may be used as a garnish if preferred.
13. Keep warm before serving.

Nutrition Information (per serving, excluding noodles or rice):

Calories: 350

Total Fat: 20g

Cholesterol: 90mg

Sodium: 400mg

Total Carbohydrates: 10g

Dietary Fiber: 1g

Sugars: 3g

Protein: 30g

<u>BBQ Pulled Pork Sandwiches</u>

Prep Time: 15 minutes

Cook Time: 6-8 hours (slow cooker) or 2-3 hours (oven)

Servings: 6-8

Ingredients:

- 3-4 lbs. pork shoulder or butt, trimmed of excess fat
- Salt and pepper to taste
- 1 onion, sliced
- 1 cup of barbecue sauce
- ½ cup of chicken broth or water
- Hamburger buns or sandwich rolls
- Coleslaw (optional, for serving)

Instructions:

1. Add salt and pepper to the pork shoulder or butt.
2. Lay the sliced onion on the bottom of a roasting pan or slow cooker.
3. After you've layered the onions, add the seasoned pork.
4. Combine the barbecue sauce with the chicken broth or water in a basin. Spoon the sauce over the meat.
5. Put the pork in a slow cooker and set the temperature to low for 6-8 hours, or bake it at 325°F (160°C) for 2-3 hours, or until it's soft and easily shredded with a fork.
6. Use two forks to shred the pork once it's done.
7. Top the pulled pork with coleslaw and serve on sandwich rolls or hamburger buns.

Nutrition Information (per serving, without coleslaw):

Calories: 400

Total Fat: 20g

Cholesterol: 120mg

Sodium: 600mg

Total Carbohydrates: 20g

Dietary Fiber: 1g

Sugars: 10g

Protein: 30g

Mongolian Beef

Prep Time: 15 minutes

Cook Time: 15 minutes

Servings: 4

Ingredients:

- 1 lb. flank steak, thinly sliced against the grain
- Salt and pepper to taste
- 2 **tbsp.** cornstarch
- 2 **tbsp.** vegetable oil
- 3 cloves garlic, minced
- 1 **tsp** grated ginger
- ½ cup of soy sauce
- ¼ cup of water
- ¼ cup of brown sugar
- 2 green onions, sliced
- Cooked rice for serving
- Sesame seeds for garnish

Instructions:

1. Sprinkle some salt and pepper on the flank steak that has been thinly cut. Coat well with cornstarch.
2. In a big wok or pan set over medium-high heat, warm the vegetable oil.
3. Layer the skillet with the cut flank steak. After sear-frying one side for one or two minutes without stirring, continue to stir-fry for another or two minutes until golden.
4. Take the meat out of the pan and put it aside.
5. Garlic and ginger, when minced, go into the same pan. Simmer for 30 seconds, or until the aroma wafts through.
6. Toss in the brown sugar, water, and soy sauce in the pan. Once the sugar has dissolved, stir.
7. Throw the cooked meat back into the pan and give it a good stir to distribute the sauce.
8. The sauce needs to thicken and coat the steak, so cook it for another two or three minutes.
9. Add sliced green onions and mix well.
10. Top cooked rice with the Mongolian meat and serve hot.
11. If you want, you may top it up with sesame seeds.

Nutrition Information:

Calories: 350

Total Fat: 15g

Cholesterol: 60mg

Sodium: 1000mg

Total Carbohydrates: 20g

Dietary Fiber: 1g

Sugars: 15g

Protein: 30g

Skinny Beef Enchiladas

Prep Time: 20 minutes

Cook Time: 25 minutes

Servings: 4-6

Ingredients:

- 1 lb. lean ground beef
- 1 onion, chopped
- 2 cloves garlic, minced
- 1 bell pepper, chopped
- 1 **tsp** ground cumin
- 1 **tsp** chili powder
- Salt and pepper to taste
- 1 (15 oz) can black beans, drained and rinsed
- 1 cup of salsa, divided
- 1 cup of shredded reduced-fat Mexican blend cheese, divided
- 8 whole wheat tortillas (8-inch size)
- Chopped fresh cilantro for garnish (optional)
- Sliced avocado for serving (optional)

- Greek yogurt or low-fat sour cream for serving (optional)

Instructions:

1. Bake at 375 degrees Fahrenheit (190 degrees Celsius). Grease a baking dish that measures 9 by 13 inches.
2. Brown the ground beef in a large pan over medium heat. Take off any extra fat.
3. Sauté the ground beef in a pan with minced garlic, chopped onion, and bell pepper. After three or four minutes of cooking, the veggies should be tender.
4. Add pepper, chili powder, salt, and ground cumin; stir to combine. After one minute, cook no more.
5. Incorporate black beans and half a cup of salsa into the pan. Toss to mix and heat for two or three minutes, or until done.
6. Stop the heat under the skillet. Add half a cup of shredded cheese and mix well.
7. Roll up each tortilla with a spoonful of the beef mixture, then lay seam side down in the baking dish that

you had previously prepared.

8. Place the enchiladas on a platter and top with the leftover salsa. Top with the rest of the crumbled cheese.
9. After 20 to 25 minutes of preheating the oven, cover the baking dish with foil and bake until the cheese melts and bubbles.
10. If you want, you may top it off with some chopped fresh cilantro. Top with sliced avocado and serve hot. For a tangy side, try Greek yogurt or low-fat sour cream.

Nutrition Information (per serving, assuming 6 servings):

Calories: 380

Total Fat: 12g

Cholesterol: 45mg

Sodium: 800mg

Total Carbohydrates: 40g

Dietary Fiber: 8g

Sugars: 4g

Protein: 28g

Pork Carnitas Tacos

Prep Time: 20 minutes

Cook Time: 4 hours (slow cooker) or 2 hours (oven)

Servings: 6-8

Ingredients:

- 3 lbs. pork shoulder, trimmed and cut into chunks
- Salt and pepper to taste
- 1 tbsp. olive oil
- 1 onion, chopped
- 4 cloves garlic, minced
- 1 **tsp** ground cumin
- 1 **tsp** dried oregano
- 1 **tsp** chili powder
- ½ **tsp** smoked paprika
- ½ **tsp** ground coriander
- ½ **tsp** cinnamon
- 1 cup of chicken broth
- Juice of 2 limes
- Corn or flour tortillas for serving
- Chopped fresh cilantro for garnish
- Sliced radishes for garnish
- Lime wedges for serving

Instructions:

1. Add salt and pepper to the pork shoulder portions.
2. A big skillet with olive oil in it should be heated over medium-high heat. If you need to, brown the pork pieces in batches and be sure

to flip them over. Place the meat that has been browned in a slow cooker.

3. Toss in the minced garlic and diced onion in the same pan. Sauté until tender, which should take around three to four minutes.
4. Then, combine the cinnamon, powdered coriander, chili powder, dried oregano, and ground cumin. Continue cooking for one more minute or until the aroma wafts into the air.
5. Before adding the meat to the slow cooker, stir in the onion and spice combination.
6. Before placing the pork in the slow cooker, pour the chicken stock and lime juice over it.
7. To make pork that readily shreds, cover and simmer for 6-8 hours on low heat or 4 hours on high heat.
8. The pork should be taken out of the slow cooker after it is done and shredded with two forks.
9. To thicken and decrease the cooking liquid, you may pour it from the slow cooker into a saucepan and heat it, if you choose.
10. The shredded pork caritas are best served in tortillas with a little lime juice, sliced radishes, and chopped fresh cilantro on top. If you'd like, you may drizzle the decreased cooking liquid on top.

Nutrition Information (per serving, assuming 8 servings):

Calories: 320

Total Fat: 20g

Cholesterol: 90mg

Sodium: 600mg

Total Carbohydrates: 4g

Dietary Fiber: 1g

Sugars: 1g

Protein: 30g

Beef and Cabbage Stir-Fry

Prep Time: 15 minutes

Cook Time: 15 minutes

Servings: 4

Ingredients:

- 1 lb. beef sirloin, thinly sliced
- Salt and pepper to taste

- 2 **tbsp.** soy sauce
- 1 tbsp. oyster sauce
- 1 tbsp. sesame oil
- 2 **tbsp.** vegetable oil
- 3 cloves garlic, minced
- 1 **tsp** grated ginger
- 4 cups of shredded cabbage
- 1 carrot, julienned
- 1 bell pepper, thinly sliced
- Cooked rice or noodles for serving
- Chopped green onions for garnish (optional)
- Sesame seeds for garnish (optional)

Instructions:

1. Add salt and pepper to the pork shoulder portions.
2. A big skillet with olive oil in it should be heated over medium-high heat. If you need to, brown the pork pieces in batches and be sure to flip them over. Place the meat that has been browned in a slow cooker.
3. Toss in the minced garlic and diced onion in the same pan. Sauté until tender, which should take around three to four minutes.
4. Then, combine the cinnamon, powdered coriander, chili powder, dried oregano, and ground cumin. Continue cooking for one more minute or until the aroma wafts into the air.
5. Before adding the meat to the slow cooker, stir in the onion and spice combination.
6. Before placing the pork in the slow cooker, pour the chicken stock and lime juice over it.
7. To make pork that readily shreds, cover and simmer for 6-8 hours on low heat or 4 hours on high heat.
8. The pork should be taken out of the slow cooker after it is done and shredded with two forks.
9. To thicken and decrease the cooking liquid, you may pour it from the slow cooker into a saucepan and heat it, if you choose.
10. The shredded pork caritas are best served in tortillas with a little lime juice, sliced radishes, and chopped fresh cilantro on top. If you'd like, you may drizzle the decreased cooking liquid on top.

Nutrition Information (per

serving, excluding rice or noodles):

Calories: 320

Total Fat: 20g

Cholesterol: 60mg

Sodium: 700mg

Total Carbohydrates: 10g

Dietary Fiber: 3g

Sugars: 4g

Protein: 25g

Italian Sausage and Peppers

Prep Time: 10 minutes

Cook Time: 25 minutes

Servings: 4

Ingredients:

- 4 Italian sausages (sweet or hot), sliced
- 1 tbsp. olive oil
- 1 onion, sliced
- 2 bell peppers, sliced (assorted colors)
- 2 cloves garlic, minced
- 1 **tsp** dried oregano
- 1 **tsp** dried basil
- Salt and pepper to taste
- 1 (14.5 oz) can diced tomatoes
- Cooked pasta or crusty bread for serving
- Grated Parmesan cheese for garnish (optional)
- Chopped fresh parsley for garnish (optional)

Instructions:

1. A big skillet with olive oil in it should be heated over medium-high heat.
2. Toss in some sliced Italian sausages and sear them until they're golden brown. Take it off the heat and put it aside.
3. Toss in the bell peppers and chopped onion in the same pan. Just give it a quick 5-minute cook till it's mushy.
4. In a pan, combine minced garlic, dried oregano and basil, salt, and pepper. Continue cooking for one more minute or until the aroma wafts into the air.
5. Put the Italian sausages back in the pan once they've cooked.
6. Top the pepper and sausage combination with chopped tomatoes and their juices. Combine by stirring.

7. After the heat is turned down to low, cover and simmer, stirring regularly, for 15 minutes.
8. Over cooked spaghetti or over crusty bread, serve the Italian sausage and peppers hot.
9. If you'd like, you may top it up with some grated Parmesan and chopped fresh parsley.

Nutrition Information (per serving, excluding pasta or bread):

Calories: 380

Total Fat: 25g

Cholesterol: 60mg

Sodium: 800mg

Total Carbohydrates: 12g

Dietary Fiber: 3g

Sugars: 6g

Protein: 25g

Beef and Vegetable Lo Mein

Prep Time: 15 minutes

Cook Time: 15 minutes

Servings: 4

Ingredients:

- 8 oz. lo Mein noodles or spaghetti
- 1 lb. flank steak, thinly sliced against the grain
- 2 **tbsp.** soy sauce
- 1 tbsp. oyster sauce
- 1 tbsp. hoisin sauce
- 1 **tsp** sesame oil
- 2 **tbsp.** vegetable oil, divided
- 3 cloves garlic, minced
- 1 **tsp** grated ginger
- 1 onion, sliced
- 1 bell pepper, thinly sliced
- 1 carrot, julienned
- 1 cup of broccoli florets
- 1 cup of snap peas
- Salt and pepper to taste
- 2 green onions, sliced for garnish

Instructions:

1. Make sure to follow the package directions while cooking the lo Mein noodles. After draining, put away.
2. Combine the four sauces (soy, oyster, hoisin, and sesame oil) in a basin. Put aside.
3. Turn up the heat to high in a big wok or pan and add 1 tbsp. of vegetable oil.

4. Sauté the flank steak slices in a pan for two or three minutes, or until they begin to brown. Take it off the heat and put it aside.
5. Get the other tbsp. of vegetable oil hot in the same pan.
6. Toss in the grated ginger and minced garlic and stir-fry for 30 seconds, or until fragrant.
7. Sauté the bell pepper, onion, carrot, snap peas, and broccoli florets until they are tender. Cook, stirring occasionally, for three to four minutes, or until crisp-tender.
8. Put the steak back in the pan when it has cooked.
9. Top the steak and veggies with the sauce mixture. After mixing well, heat until heated through.
10. Sauté the lo Mein noodles when they're done. Coat everything evenly with the sauce by tossing it together.
11. Add salt and pepper according to your preference.
12. Slice some green onions and place them on top before serving.

Nutrition Information (per serving):

Calories: 450

Total Fat: 15g

Cholesterol: 60mg

Sodium: 800mg

Total Carbohydrates: 50g

Dietary Fiber: 5g

Sugars: 6g

Protein: 30g

Pork and Veggie Kebabs

Prep Time: 20 minutes

Cook Time: 15 minutes

Servings: 4

Ingredients:

- 1 lb. pork tenderloin, cut into cubes
- 1 bell pepper, cut into chunks
- 1 onion, cut into chunks
- 1 zucchini, sliced
- 1 cup of cherry tomatoes
- 8 wooden skewers, soaked in water for 30 minutes
- Salt and pepper to taste
- 2 **tbsp.** olive oil
- 2 **tbsp.** soy sauce
- 1 tbsp. honey

- 1 tbsp. Dijon mustard
- 1 **tsp** minced garlic
- 1 **tsp** dried oregano
- 1 **tsp** dried thyme

Instructions:

1. Turn the grill on high heat and let it heat up.
2. Stuff the soaked wooden skewers with a variety of ingredients, switching between pork cubes, bell pepper pieces, onion chunks, zucchini slices, and cherry tomatoes.
3. Add pepper and salt to taste to the kebabs.
4. Create the marinade by whisking together the following ingredients in a small bowl: olive oil, soy sauce, honey, Dijon mustard, minced garlic, dried oregano, and dried thyme.
5. Coat the kebabs equally with the marinade by brushing it on them.
6. Before you put the kebabs on the grill, make sure it's hot. Cook for 10 to 12 minutes, flipping once, or until the pork is done and the veggies are soft.
7. After taking the kebabs from the grill, give them a few minutes to rest before cutting into them.
8. Warm up some rice or salad and serve the pork and vegetable kebabs.

Nutrition Information (per serving):

Calories: 320

Total Fat: 10g

Cholesterol: 75mg

Sodium: 450mg

Total Carbohydrates: 20g

Dietary Fiber: 3g

Sugars: 10g

Protein: 35g

DESSERT AND SNACK

Skinny Apple Crisp

Prep Time: 15 minutes

Cook Time: 35 minutes

Servings: 6

Ingredients:

- 4 cups of apples, peeled, cored, and sliced (such as Granny Smith)
- 1 tbsp. lemon juice
- ¼ cup of granulated sugar
- 1 **tsp** ground cinnamon
- ¼ **tsp** ground nutmeg
- ½ cup of old-fashioned oats
- ¼ cup of whole wheat flour
- ¼ cup of packed brown sugar
- 2 **tbsp.** unsalted butter, melted
- 2 **tbsp.** chopped walnuts or pecans (optional)
- Cooking spray

Instructions:

1. Bake at 375 degrees Fahrenheit (190 degrees Celsius). Spray a baking dish that is 8 inches square with cooking spray.
2. Toss the sliced apples in a large basin with the granulated sugar, cinnamon, nutmeg, and lemon juice until they are evenly covered. Evenly distribute the apple mixture into the baking dish that has been preheated.
3. Oleo, whole wheat flour, brown sugar, melted butter, and chopped nuts (if used) should all be combined in the same bowl. Work the mixture until it becomes a crumbly texture.
4. Divide the oat mixture among the apples in the baking dish and sprinkle it evenly.
5. To get a golden brown topping and soft apples, bake in a preheated oven for 30–35 minutes.
6. After taking it out of the oven, let it a few minutes to cool down before cutting into it.
7. Warm up some slim apple crisp and top it with low-fat vanilla ice cream or Greek yogurt, if you want.

Nutrition Information (per serving):

Calories: 160

Total Fat: 4.5g

Cholesterol: 8mg

Sodium: 25mg

Total Carbohydrates: 30g

Dietary Fiber: 3g

Sugars: 20g

Protein: 2g

Key Lime Pie Yogurt Parfait

Prep Time: 10 minutes

Cook Time: None

Servings: 2

Ingredients:

- 1 cup of plain Greek yogurt
- Zest of 1 lime
- 2 **tbsp.** fresh lime juice
- 2 **tbsp.** honey or maple syrup
- ½ cup of graham cracker crumbs
- 1 tbsp. unsalted butter, melted
- Whipped cream for topping (optional)
- Lime slices for garnish (optional)

Instructions:

1. The zest and juice of one lime, together with some honey or maple syrup, and some Greek yogurt should be mixed well in a small bowl. Put aside.
2. Melt the butter in a separate dish and whisk in the graham cracker crumbs until the crumbs are uniformly coated.
3. In serving bowls or glasses, alternate layers of graham cracker crumbs and lime yogurt, working your way around the bowls or glasses.
4. After you've used all of the ingredients, repeat the steps one more time, ending with a layer of crushed graham crackers.
5. Garnish each parfait with a lime slice and a dollop of whipped cream, if desired.
6. Keep the key lime pie yogurt parfaits in the fridge until serving time, or serve them right away.

Nutrition Information (per serving):

Calories: 280

Total Fat: 11g

Cholesterol: 20mg

Sodium: 160mg

Total Carbohydrates: 37g

Dietary Fiber: 2g

Sugars: 24g

Protein: 12g

Chocolate Zucchini Bread

Prep Time: 15 minutes

Cook Time: 50-60 minutes

Servings: 12

Ingredients:

- 1-½ cups of grated zucchini (about 1 medium zucchini)
- 1 cup of all-purpose flour
- ½ cup of unsweetened cocoa powder
- 1 **tsp** baking powder
- ½ **tsp** baking soda
- ½ **tsp** salt
- ½ **tsp** ground cinnamon
- ¼ cup of vegetable oil
- ½ cup of granulated sugar
- ½ cup of packed brown sugar
- 2 large eggs
- 1 **tsp** vanilla extract
- ½ cup of chocolate chips (optional)

Instructions:

1. Set the oven temperature to 350°F, or 175°C. Preheat a loaf pan that measures 9 by 5 inches.
2. Squeeze off any extra moisture from the shredded zucchini using a clean kitchen towel.
3. Flour, cocoa powder, baking soda, salt, cinnamon, and baking powder should be whipped together in a big basin.
4. Blend the eggs, brown sugar, granulated sugar, vegetable oil, and vanilla essence in a separate dish.
5. Just mix the dry and wet components by stirring them together.
6. After grating the zucchini, stir in the chocolate chips (if using) and mix till combined.
7. Evenly distribute the batter into the loaf pan that has been prepared.
8. Fifty to sixty minutes into the preheated oven, or until a toothpick inserted in the middle comes out clean.
9. The bread needs 10 minutes to cool in the pan after taking it out of the oven, and then it may be transferred to a wire rack to finish cooling.
10. Cut and serve when it has cooled.

Nutrition Information (per serving):

Calories: 200

Total Fat: 8g

Cholesterol: 30mg

Sodium: 200mg

Total Carbohydrates: 31g

Dietary Fiber: 2g

Sugars: 19g

Protein: 3g

<u>Lemon Poppy Seed Muffins</u>

Prep Time: 15 minutes

Cook Time: 18-20 minutes

Servings: 12

Ingredients:

- 2 cups of all-purpose flour
- 3/4 cup of granulated sugar
- 2 **tbsp.** poppy seeds
- 2 **tsp** baking powder
- ½ **tsp** baking soda
- ¼ **tsp** salt
- Zest of 2 lemons
- 3/4 cup of buttermilk
- 1/3 cup of vegetable oil
- 2 large eggs
- 2 **tbsp.** fresh lemon juice
- 1 **tsp** vanilla extract

Instructions:

1. Bake at 375 degrees Fahrenheit (190 degrees Celsius). Grease or line a 12-cup muffin pan with paper liners.
2. Flour, sugar, poppy seeds, baking soda, salt, lemon zest, and baking powder should all be whisked together in a big basin.
3. Combine the eggs, buttermilk, vegetable oil, lemon juice, and vanilla extract in a separate dish and whisk until smooth.
4. Stir the dry ingredients into the wet ones until they are barely mixed. The batter should have some lumps in it, so be careful not to overmix.
5. Fill up each of the muffin tins about two-thirds of the way to the top with batter.
6. Poke a toothpick into the middle of each muffin and bake for 18 to 20 minutes, or until the pick comes out clean.
7. When the muffins have cooled for 5 minutes in the pan, take them out of the oven and set them on a wire rack to finish cooling.
8. Serve and savor when it has cooled.

Nutrition Information (per muffin):

Calories: 200

Total Fat: 8g

Cholesterol: 35mg

Sodium: 180mg

Total Carbohydrates: 29g

Dietary Fiber: 1g

Sugars: 14g

Protein: 3g

Skinny Banana Bread

Prep Time: 15 minutes

Cook Time: 50-60 minutes

Servings: 12

Ingredients:

- 3 ripe bananas, mashed
- 1/3 cup of unsweetened applesauce
- ¼ cup of plain Greek yogurt
- ¼ cup of honey or maple syrup
- 1 **tsp** vanilla extract
- 1 ½ cups of whole wheat flour
- 1 **tsp** baking powder
- ½ **tsp** baking soda
- ½ **tsp** salt
- ½ **tsp** ground cinnamon
- Optional: ¼ cup of chopped nuts (such as walnuts or pecans)

Instructions:

1. Set the oven temperature to 350°F, or 175°C. Preheat a loaf pan that measures 9 by 5 inches.
2. Whisk together the mashed bananas, applesauce, Greek yoghurt, honey (or maple syrup), and vanilla extract in a large mixing dish. Blend everything together.
3. In another bowl, combine the whole wheat flour, baking soda, salt, cinnamon powder, baking powder, and whisk until well combined.
4. Stirring constantly, add the dry mixture to the wet mixture little by little until just mixed. Stir gently.
5. Carefully incorporate chopped nuts into the batter if using.
6. Evenly distribute the batter into the loaf pan that has been prepared.
7. Fifty to sixty minutes into the preheated oven, or until a toothpick inserted in the middle comes out clean.
8. After 10 minutes of cooling in the pan, take the pan out

of the oven and set the banana bread on a wire rack to finish cooling.
9. Cut and serve when it has cooled.

Nutrition Information (per serving):

Calories: 120

Total Fat: 1g

Cholesterol: 0mg

Sodium: 160mg

Total Carbohydrates: 27g

Dietary Fiber: 3g

Sugars: 10g

Protein: 3g

Cucumber Sandwiches with Hummus

Prep Time: 10 minutes

Cook Time: None

Servings: 4

Ingredients:

- 8 slices whole grain bread
- 1 large cucumber, thinly sliced
- ½ cup of hummus (store-bought or homemade)
- ¼ cup of fresh basil leaves
- Salt and pepper to taste

Instructions:

1. Divide the hummus among the whole grain bread slices and spread it out equally.
2. Divide the bread in half and top each piece with cucumber slices.
3. Add salt and pepper to the cucumbers according to your taste.
4. Garniture: fresh basil leaves.
5. Fill up the sandwiches with the rest of the bread pieces.
6. Slice the sandwiches in half or quarters and remove the crusts if you want.
7. Sandwiches may be served right away or carefully wrapped in plastic and chilled until needed.

Nutrition Information (per serving, based on 2 sandwiches):

Calories: 270

Total Fat: 7g

Cholesterol: 0mg

Sodium: 480mg

Total Carbohydrates: 41g

Dietary Fiber: 7g

Sugars: 5g

Protein: 12g

Frozen Grapes

Prep Time: 5 minutes

Cook Time: 0 minutes

Servings: Variable

Ingredients:

- Fresh grapes (any variety)

Instructions:

1. Gently rinse the grapes under cold water and then dry them with a paper towel.
2. After lining a baking sheet with parchment paper or a silicone mat, spread the grapes out in a single layer.
3. After 2 hours, or when the grapes are fully frozen, transfer the baking sheet to the freezer.
4. After the grapes have frozen, store them in an airtight container or freezer bag.
5. As a cool and nutritious snack, serve the grapes directly from the freezer.

Nutrition Information (per serving, approximately 1 cup of):

Calories: 60

Total Fat: 0g

Cholesterol: 0mg

Sodium: 0mg

Total Carbohydrates: 15g

Dietary Fiber: 1g

Sugars: 15g

Protein: 1g

Skinny Raspberry Sorbet

Prep Time: 5 minutes

Cook Time: 0 minutes

Chilling Time: 2-3 hours

Servings: 4

Ingredients:

- 3 cups of frozen raspberries
- ¼ cup of honey or maple syrup
- 2 **tbsp.** fresh lemon juice
- ¼ cup of water (if needed)

Instructions:

1. Put the fresh lemon juice, honey (or maple syrup), and frozen raspberries into a blender or food processor.
2. While scraping down the sides of the bowl as necessary, blend the mixture until it becomes smooth and creamy. If you find that the mixture is too thick to

combine, slowly add **tbsp.** of water until it achieves the consistency you prefer.

3. Smooth up the sorbet mixture and pour it into a shallow dish or container.
4. Place a cover or plastic wrap on top of the dish or container and place in the freezer for two to three hours, or until the sorbet is solid.
5. Sorbet needs a few minutes to soften at room temperature before serving.
6. Quickly serve the slender raspberry sorbet by scooping it into cones or bowls.

Nutrition Information (per serving): Calories: 70, Total Fat: 0g, Cholesterol: 0mg, Sodium: 0mg, Total Carbohydrates: 18g, Dietary Fiber: 4g, Sugars: 12g, Protein: 1g

<u>Mini Cheesecake Bites</u>

Prep Time: 20 minutes

Cook Time: 15 minutes

Chilling Time: 2 hours

Servings: 24 mini cheesecake bites

Ingredients:

- 1 cup of graham cracker crumbs
- 2 **tbsp.** granulated sugar
- 3 **tbsp.** unsalted butter, melted
- 8 oz. cream cheese, softened
- ¼ cup of sour cream
- ¼ cup of granulated sugar
- 1 large egg
- 1 **tsp** vanilla extract
- Fresh berries or fruit preserves for topping (optional)

Instructions:

1. Set the oven temperature to 350°F, or 175°C. Place paper liners into a 24-cup mini muffin pan.
2. Mix the sugar, melted butter, and graham cracker crumbs in a small bowl. Blend everything together.
3. Using the back of a spoon, press about 1 spoonful of the graham cracker mixture into the base of each muffin cup.
4. To make the cream cheese mixture, in a bowl, combine the sour cream, sugar, egg, and vanilla extract. Beat until combined.
5. Divide the cream cheese mixture equally among the muffin pan cups lined with

graham cracker crusts and fill each one almost to the top with the mixture.

6. The cheesecake filling should be set after 12–15 minutes in a preheated oven.
7. After taking the mini cheesecakes out of the oven, set them aside to cool for 10 minutes in the muffin pan.
8. Once cooled, place the miniature cheesecakes on a wire rack and chill in the fridge for at least two hours, or until totally cooled.
9. As a finishing touch, you may garnish each individual little cheesecake with a few berries or a small dollop of fruit preserves before serving.

Nutrition Information (per serving): Calories: 90, Total Fat: 6g, Cholesterol: 25mg, Sodium: 70mg, Total Carbohydrates: 7g, Sugars: 5g, Protein: 1g

Carrot Cake Energy Balls

Prep Time: 15 minutes

Chilling Time: 30 minutes

Servings: 12 energy balls

Ingredients:

- 1 cup of rolled oats
- ½ cup of shredded carrots
- ¼ cup of chopped walnuts or pecans
- ¼ cup of raisins or dried cranberries
- 2 **tbsp.** honey or maple syrup
- 1 tbsp. coconut oil, melted
- ½ **tsp** ground cinnamon
- ¼ **tsp** ground nutmeg
- Pinch of salt
- Shredded coconut or additional chopped nuts for coating (optional)

Instructions:

1. Toss the rolled oats, chopped nuts, shredded carrots, honey (or maple syrup), melted coconut oil, crushed cinnamon, powdered nutmeg, and a bit of salt into a food processor. Add the raisins or dried cranberries and mix well.
2. Once everything is incorporated and begins to stick together, pulse the mixture.
3. Divide the mixture into 12 energy balls using your hands. Each ball should have around 1 tbsp. of the ingredients.

4. Energy balls may be coated with shredded coconut or extra chopped nuts if preferred.
5. After 30 minutes in the fridge, or until they are hard, transfer the energy balls to a parchment-lined baking sheet.
6. Put the carrot cake energy balls in the fridge until they're ready to eat once they've cooled.

Nutrition Information (per serving): Calories: 90, Total Fat: 4g, Cholesterol: 0mg, Sodium: 10mg, Total Carbohydrates: 14g, Sugars: 7g, Protein: 2g, these recipes offer

Chocolate Chip Cookie Dough Dip

Prep Time: 10 minutes

Cook Time: 0 minutes

Servings: 8

Ingredients:

- 1 (15 oz.) can chickpeas, drained and rinsed
- ¼ cup of almond butter or peanut butter
- ¼ cup of honey or maple syrup
- 1 tsp vanilla extract
- ¼ **tsp** salt
- ¼ cup of mini chocolate chips

Instructions:

1. Toss the chickpeas with the peanut or almond butter, honey or maple syrup, vanilla extract, and salt in a food processor.
2. Scrape down the edges of the bowl as required to ensure a smooth and creamy texture as you process.
3. Gather the ingredients in a dish and gently incorporate the small chocolate chips.
4. Dip some fruit, pretzels, or graham crackers into the chocolate chip cookie dough and serve it hot.
5. Put any leftovers in a sealed jar and refrigerate for no more than three days.

Nutrition Information (per serving): Calories: 160, Total Fat: 6g, Cholesterol: 0mg, Sodium: 110mg, Total Carbohydrates: 24g, Dietary Fiber: 4g, Sugars: 14g, Protein: 5g

Skinny Blueberry Muffins

Prep Time: 10 minutes

Cook Time: 20 minutes

Servings: 12 muffins

Ingredients:

- 1-½ cups of whole wheat flour
- ½ cup of old-fashioned oats
- ½ cup of granulated sugar or sweetener of choice
- 2 **tsp** baking powder
- ½ **tsp** baking soda
- ¼ **tsp** salt
- ½ cup of unsweetened applesauce
- ½ cup of non-fat Greek yogurt
- ¼ cup of almond milk or skim milk
- 1 large egg
- 1 **tsp** vanilla extract
- 1 cup of fresh or frozen blueberries

Instructions:

1. Bake at 375 degrees Fahrenheit (190 degrees Celsius). Grease or line a 12-cup muffin pan with paper liners.
2. Everything you need for this recipe is in a big bowl: whole wheat flour, oats, sugar, baking soda, baking powder, and salt. Whisk to combine.
3. Mix the almond milk, applesauce, Greek yogurt, egg, and vanilla extract in a separate dish. Blend everything together.
4. Stir the dry ingredients into the wet ones until they are barely mixed. Stir gently.
5. Toss the blueberries gently into the batter until they are equally distributed.
6. Fill up each of the muffin tins about two-thirds of the way to the top with batter.
7. Poke a toothpick into the middle of each muffin and bake for 18 to 20 minutes, or until the pick comes out clean.
8. When the muffins have cooled for 5 minutes in the pan, take them out of the oven and set them on a wire rack to finish cooling.
9. Serve and savor when it has cooled.

Nutrition Information (per muffin): Calories: 140, Total Fat: 1.5g, Cholesterol: 15mg, Sodium: 180mg, Total Carbohydrates: 28g,

Dietary Fiber: 3g, Sugars: 12g, Protein: 4g

Strawberry Banana Popsicles

Prep Time: 10 minutes

Freezing Time: 4 hours

Servings: 6 popsicles

Ingredients:

- 1 cup of sliced strawberries
- 1 ripe banana
- ½ cup of plain Greek yogurt
- 2 **tbsp.** honey or maple syrup
- ½ **tsp** vanilla extract

Instructions:

1. Throw in some sliced strawberries, a banana, some Greek yogurt, some honey (or maple syrup), and some vanilla essence, and pulse until smooth.
2. Combine all ingredients and blend until smooth.
3. Fill up all of the Popsicle molds with the mixture.
4. Fill the molds with Popsicle sticks.
5. Freeze the Popsicle molds for a minimum of four hours, or until they solidify.
6. Popsicles should be served shortly after being removed from their molds once frozen.
7. If you're having problems releasing the popsicles from their molds, try running warm water over their exteriors.

Nutrition Information (per Popsicle): Calories: 50, Total Fat: 0g, Cholesterol: 0mg, Sodium: 5mg, Total Carbohydrates: 11g, Dietary Fiber: 1g, Sugars: 8g, Protein: 2g

Peanut Butter

Prep Time: 5 minutes

Cook Time: None

Servings: Variable

Ingredients:

- 1 cup of unsalted peanuts (you can also use roasted peanuts for more flavor)
- 1-2 **tbsp.** honey or maple syrup (optional)
- Pinch of salt (optional)

Instructions:

1. Put the peanuts into a blender.

2. Once the peanuts begin to clump together, process for another minute or two, stopping to scrape down the sides as needed.
3. Honey, maple syrup, or a touch of salt may be added if preferred.
4. The peanut butter should be processed for a further one to two minutes, or until it achieves the consistency you like.
5. Once the peanut butter is ready, transfer it to an airtight container or jar.
6. You may keep the peanut butter in the fridge for a maximum of two weeks.

Nutrition Information (per 2 **tbsp.**): Calories: 180, Total Fat: 15g, Cholesterol: 0mg, Sodium: 0mg, Total Carbohydrates: 6g

Dietary Fiber: 2g, Sugars: 2g, Protein: 8g

Conclusion: _

Thanks for reading all the way through "The Complete Zero Point Weight Loss Cookbook!" You should now have a better idea of how zero-point foods can affect your weight loss efforts. This cookbook isn't just a collection of recipes; it's also meant to provide ideas for a healthier lifestyle that is enjoyable and sustainable.

Embracing a Healthier Lifestyle

This cookbook's recipes and meal plans show that eating healthy doesn't have to be boring or stressful. Lots of different tastes and textures are available in zero-point foods, so you can still eat tasty meals while sticking to your weight loss goals. Your daily intake of these foods is a big step toward a healthier lifestyle.

Key Takeaways

Flexibility and freedom: Zero-point foods give you a versatile framework that lets you enjoy a wide range of foods without having to carefully count calories. This freedom makes dieting less stressful and anxious.

Nutrient-Dense Options: Eating a lot of zero-point foods will make sure that your diet is full of important nutrients, which is important for your mental and physical health. For fewer unhealthy snacks, these foods make you feel full and satisfied.

Sustainable Habits: The zero point approach helps people form longer-lasting eating habits. Long-term success at keeping a healthy weight comes from choosing foods that are both healthy and low in calories.

The Road Ahead for You

The path to losing weight and improving your health is unique to each person and is full of both struggles and successes. Remember that advancement doesn't always happen in a straight line, and setbacks are normal parts of the process. You can use the tools and recipes in this cookbook as a starting point for your journey, but feel free to change and try new things based on your own individual needs and preferences.

Help yourself while staying focused on your goals. Any small wins should be celebrated, and short-term setbacks shouldn't get you down. Moving toward healthier eating is a win in and of itself.

Lastly,

Beyond a book of recipes, "The Complete Zero Point Weight Loss Cookbook" is a guide to a healthier, happier you. You can change your relationship with food and make lasting, positive changes in your life by adopting the zero point philosophy.

After reading this cookbook, we hope you're motivated to cook more, eat better, and enjoy the process of finding new, healthy recipes. While you're working to improve your health, remember that you have all the information and tools you need to make daily healthy decisions.

We appreciate you letting us help you lose weight. Wishing you success, good health, and happiness! Savor the process, enjoy the tasty recipes, and commit to living a zero-point lifestyle. Lots of luck cooking!

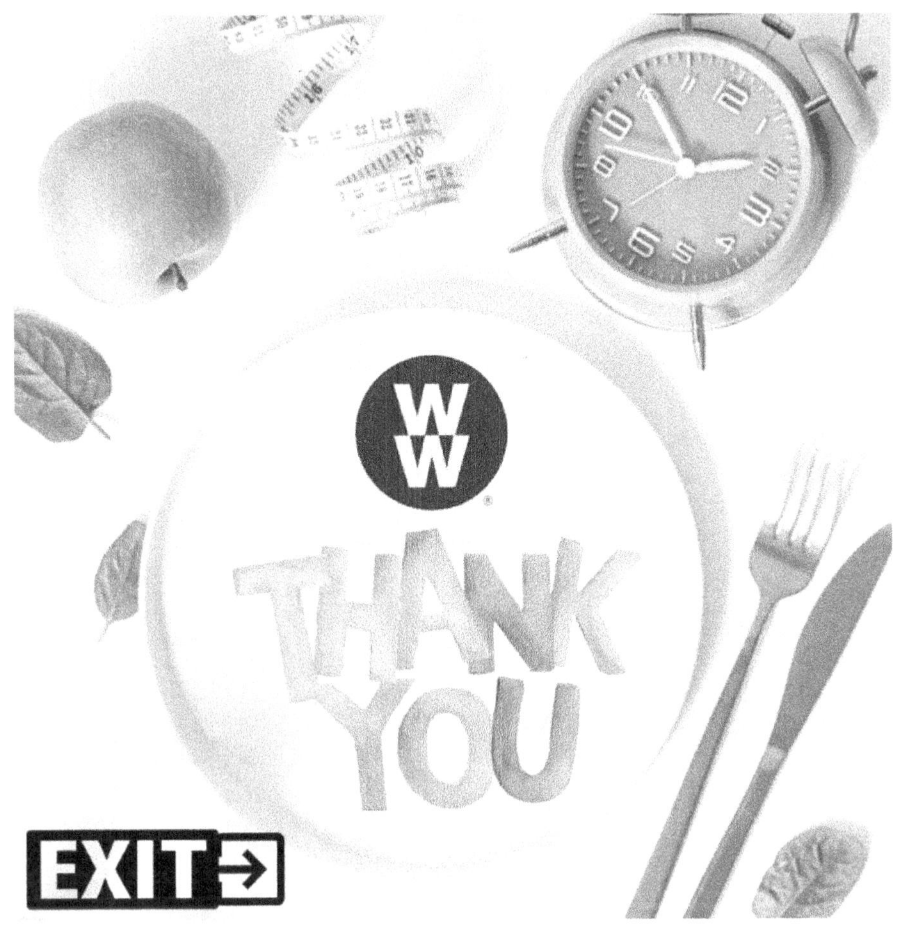
WW
THANK YOU
EXIT →

www.ingramcontent.com/pod-product-compliance
Lightning Source LLC
Chambersburg PA
CBHW081222260726
48653CB00010BB/3750